Assessment of Hearing-Impaired People

Assessment of Hearing-Impaired People

A Guide for Selecting
Psychological, Educational,
and Vocational Tests

Frank R. Zieziula, Editor

Gallaudet College Press

Published by the Gallaudet College Press
Kendall Green, Washington, DC 20002

Library of Congress Catalog Card Number 82-81439
International Standard Book Number 0-913580-80-5

All rights reserved. No part of this book may be reproduced in any form or by any method without permission in writing from the publisher.

Third Printing 1986

Copyright © 1982 by Gallaudet College
Washington, DC 20002

Gallaudet College is an equal opportunity employer/educational institution. Programs and services offered by Gallaudet College receive substantial financial support from the U.S. Department of Education.

Contributors

William Adams
Frankfurt, West Germany

Richard Arthur
Glendale, West Virginia

Susan Auerbach
Washington, D.C.

Vivian Barron
Charlotte, North Carolina

Jane Bolles
Plattsburg, New York

Veronique Bourguignon
Verrieres le Buisson, France

Barbara Bown
Riverside, California

Millie Brother
Palo Alto, California

Robert Chandler
Washington, D.C.

Barbara Cohen
New York, New York

Louise Crume
Cleveland, Ohio

Alicia Cusack-Marshall
Indianapolis, Indiana

Regina Davis
Fort Worth, Texas

Rona Denis-Siwek
Bronx, New York

Thomas Downes
Hartford, Connecticut

Susan Draper
Washington, D.C.

Lynn Eklund
Virginia, Minnesota

L'Tanya Fish
Hickory, North Carolina

Michael Gilpatrick
Bristol, Pennsylvania

Steve Glenn
Jacksonville, Florida

Wendy Gold
Brooklyn, New York

Anita Hart
Philadelphia, Pennsylvania

Sylvia Hector
Antigua, West Indies

Carolyn Hyatt
Norco, California

Bill Isham
Evanston, Illinois

George Iwashko
New York, New York

Jo Anne Jones
New Haven, Connecticut

Dorinda Jordan
Norfolk, Virginia

Maureen Kiely
Rochester, Minnesota

Jacqueline Roth Kinner
Forest Hills, New York

Toby Koritsky
Boston, Massachusetts

David Lawlor
Dover, New Hampshire

Elizabeth Loreto
Warren, Ohio

Virginia Lusebrink-Ramkomut
Pittsburgh, Pennsylvania

Wilton McMillan
Parkton, North Carolina

Marsha Micelli
Philadelphia, Pennsylvania

Eloise Molock
Cambridge, Maryland

Sue Ellen Pressman
Miami Beach, Florida

Fern Reisinger
Newark, New Jersey

Charles Riccio
Buffalo, New York

Jo Ann Robinson
Lake Village, Arkansas

Scott Robinson
Lowville, New York

Donna Sarti
Providence, Rhode Island

Pat Sells
Pueblo, Colorado

Rebecca Shearouse
Orlando, Florida

Margaret Stanton
Urbana, Illinois

Laurie Stark
Rochester, New York

Doris Stelle
Silver Spring, Maryland

Pamela Stine
St. Paul, Minnesota

Wayne Trout
Philadelphia, Pennsylvania

Catherine Wilson
Washington, D.C.

Sandra Zielinski
Pittsburgh, Pennsylvania

CONTENTS

Preface ... ix

Acknowledgments ... xiii

Introduction—Guidelines for Selecting Tests for Hearing-Impaired People ... 1

Chapter

1 Academic Achievement Tests ... 5
 Full-Range Picture Vocabulary Test ... 5
 Gates-MacGinitie Reading Tests ... 7
 Key Math Diagnostic Arithmetic Test ... 8
 Metropolitan Achievement Tests Series ... 10
 Peabody Picture Vocabulary Test ... 12
 Stanford Achievement Test—Hearing-Impaired Edition ... 14
 Verbal Language Development Scale ... 16
 Wide Range Achievement Test ... 18
 Woodcock Reading Mastery Tests ... 19

2 Communication Tests ... 21
 Denver Scale of Communication Function ... 21
 Illinois Test of Psycholinguistic Abilities (Revised) ... 23

3 Intelligence Tests ... 25
 Cattell Infant Intelligence Scale ... 25
 Columbia Mental Maturity Scale ... 27
 Denver Developmental Screening Test ... 29
 Haptic Intelligence Scale for Adult Blind ... 30
 Hiskey-Nebraska Test of Learning Aptitude ... 32
 Knox Cube Test: Arthur Revision ... 34
 Kohs Block Design Test ... 36
 Leiter International Performance Scale ... 37
 Revised Beta Examination ... 39
 Slosson Intelligence Test ... 40
 Raven's Progressive Matrices ... 42
 Stanford-Binet Intelligence Scale ... 44
 Vineland Social Maturity Scale ... 46

		Wechsler Adult Intelligence Scale—Revised	48	6	**Vocational Aptitude Tests** 87
		Wechsler Intelligence Scale for Children—Revised	50		Bennett Mechanical Comprehension Tests 87
		WISC-R Adaptation for the Deaf	52		Differential Aptitude Tests 89
Chapter					Flanagan Industrial Tests 91
4		**Personality Tests**	55		General Aptitude Test Battery ... 92
		Balthazar Scales of Adaptive Behavior I & II	55		General Clerical Test 94
		California Psychological Inventory	57		Minnesota Clerical Test 96
		California Test of Personality	58		Minnesota Rate of Manipulation Tests 97
		Devereux Adolescent Behavior Rating Scale	60		O'Conner Finger Dexterity Test and O'Conner Tweezer Dexterity Test 99
		Draw-a-Person Projective Technique (Urban's Scoring System)	61		Purdue Pegboard 100
		Handicap Problems Inventory	63		Revised Minnesota Paper Form Board Test 102
		House-Tree-Person Projective Technique (Buck Scoring System)	64	7	**Vocational Interest Tests** 105
		Meadow/Kendall Social-Emotional Assessment Inventory	66		Geist Picture Interest Inventory (Revised) 105
		Minnesota Multiphasic Personality Inventory	68		Picture Interest Exploration Survey 108
		Rorschach Method	70		Strong-Campbell Interest Inventory 109
		Tennessee Self-Concept Scale	72		Wide Range Interest and Opinion Test—Revised 111
		Thematic Apperception Test	74		
	5	**Visual Perception Tests**	77	8	**Work Evaluation Systems** 115
		Bender Visual-Motor Gestalt Test for Young Children (Koppitz Scoring System)	77		Jewish Employment and Vocational Service 115
		Benton Visual Retention Test	79		Singer Vocational Evaluation System 117
		Memory for Designs Test	81		Testing, Orientation and Work Evaluation in Rehabilitation ... 119
		Motor-Free Visual Perception Test	83		Valpar Component Work Sample Series 120
		Reitan-Indiana Neuropsychological Test Battery for Children	84		

Appendix
A **Supplementary Reading on General Aspects of Evaluating Hearing-Impaired People** 123

Appendix
B **Test Acronyms** 127

PREFACE

Two dilemmas have plagued me since I began teaching the use and interpretation of tests with hearing-impaired people at New York University some six years ago. The first dilemma is finding reading materials that answer specific questions students have about the appropriateness or inappropriateness of tests for hearing-impaired people. The second dilemma relates to creating meaningful assignments for students who have to suffer through my courses. The present text is my answer to these problems.

As for the first dilemma, the question most frequently asked by professionals who plan to work with hearing-impaired clients is, "What tests are being used in educational institutions, rehabilitation agencies, and mental health centers with this clientele?" Sometimes the question goes like this, "I use (this) test with all my other clients; can it also be used with hearing-impaired people?"

These are fair questions that deserve direct answers. For a variety of reasons (the most important of which is recent federal legislation), there is an increasing mandate to provide appropriate psychological, educational, and work-related evaluations of hearing-impaired people using standardized testing procedures. But we who specialize in this unique field have not been providing direct guidance to consumers on what test materials work best.

This text is intended to meet these consumer needs through a comprehensive review of 62 tests. The purpose is to provide the practitioner not only with "best judgments" of the usability of test instruments with hearing-impaired people but, just as importantly, to provide professionals-in-training, teachers, counselors, parents, and clients with facts and figures about the purposes and compositions of the tests themselves.

The present text is an updated and revised version of the May 1980 and September 1980 limited editions of *Psychological Tests and Deafness* in which 48 tests were reviewed.

The choice of the 62 tests in this text was mine alone. My decisions were based on two factors. First, tests well-known by most evaluators were chosen for review regardless of applicability to a hearing-impaired population. Because many of these tests are used by so many evaluators, I considered it important to review them in light of hearing-impaired people. Second, some tests were included because they have been used frequently with hearing-impaired people but are little known beyond the circle of specialists in this field.

The second dilemma—the lack of meaningful course assignments for my students—has been alleviated by asking my graduate students at Gallaudet College to write this book. Fifty-two students contributed to this work over a two-year period. The students (the majority of whom are now successful practitioners) represent the fields of school and rehabilitation counseling with hearing-impaired people. I am amazed how these young professionals can make valuable contributions to our field if we professors do not limit their thoughts, creativity, and behavior by assignments meant for the "round file" at the completion of their programs. This book testifies to that amazement.

Once the students' assignments were complete, facts and statistics were checked for accuracy and consistency. Judgments concerning use of the tests with hearing-impaired individuals were scrutinized by this editor. The students should receive any accolades for a job professionally done. I accept responsibility for omissions and poor judgments.

The text is divided into three major parts. The Introduction addresses the broad issue of selecting tests to be used with hearing-impaired people. Because it would be next to impossible to cover all tests that may be considered for use with this population, I have attempted to explicate guidelines that should be used with all tests that one may encounter.

Chapters 1 through 8 contain selected test reviews. The tests are organized by type: *academic achievement tests, communication tests, intelligence tests, personality tests, visual perception tests, vocational aptitude tests, vocational interest tests,* and *work evaluation systems.*

Two of these eight categories deserve special attention. The category of communication tests (Chapter 2) is probably new to professionals who have not worked with hearing-impaired people. These tests focus on means of communication used for daily interaction rather than audiological assessments of hearing loss. As one will note, very few tests are reviewed. This is an area of testing in which standardized test instruments are lacking or inefficient. Most people at present use self-developed rating scales of communication functioning that are unique to a particular population. These rating scales are usually weak in validity and/or reliability data. Rightly or wrongly, this is the present state of the art. More test development and empirical research must be done in this area.

Work evaluation systems (Chapter 8) is a new and exciting area in educational programming and rehabilitative services for hearing-impaired people. Traditional aptitude testing is being replaced with extensive hands-on experimentation in simulated work settings. A whole new specialty of vocational evaluation is gaining impetus in the field of rehabilitation. Because of this movement, work samples are being developed, revised, and adapted for special populations such as hearing-impaired people. The rate of progress is so fast that major changes in existing work samples systems can be expected by the time this book is in print.

For all tests, information is provided on the author, publisher, price, date of edition, general purpose of the test, description of the test, administration, special administration procedures for hearing-impaired people, age level, reliability, validity, norms, norms for hearing-impaired people, appropriateness for hearing-impaired people, range of scores, interpretation, summary of Buros Institute publications, general references, and references related to hearing-impaired people.

Prices of tests were obtained from the publishers in the spring and summer of 1981. Given our fluctuating economy, one can be assured that test prices will change on a yearly basis. The prices listed here are intended to provide the reader with ballpark figures. Check with the publisher for current price listings.

A summary of Buros Institute publications is included in each test review because of the importance of the *Mental Measurements Yearbooks* and other publications of the Buros Institute of Mental Measurements. For people unfamiliar with the late Dr. Oscar Krisen Buros's contributions to the field of testing, the *Mental Measurements Yearbooks, Tests in Print, Intelligence Tests and Reviews, Vocational Tests and Reviews, Personality Tests and Reviews,* and related publications are encyclopedias of experts' reviews on current and past tests in print. If a person wishes to utilize a specific test, I encourage him or her to go to the source of the review for a more in-depth explanation of the pros and cons of the test.*

Appendix A presents additional references on general aspects of evaluating hearing-impaired people. Appendix B alphabetically lists test acronyms used in the text. In most cases these acronyms are of my choosing and are not usually used by the test author or publisher.

Throughout the book *hearing impaired* is preferred over *deaf* or other nomenclatures to describe all individuals who are experiencing an auditory disability that may interfere with normal interaction with a variety of people and/or with the traditional communications systems and machines used in our society. The major intent of using this term, as opposed to others, is to direct the readers' attention to the fact that even a mild auditory disability should be taken into account when choosing test instruments. For those readers who prefer applying the word *deaf* to individuals experiencing auditory disabilities, I suggest this twist on a relevant proverb: "When the recommendation fits, buy it; when the recommendation doesn't seem to make sense, get a second opinion."

F.R.Z.

---

*Mental Measurements Yearbook has been published as follows: 1938 edition; 1940 edition; third edition, 1949; fourth edition, 1953; fifth edition, 1959; sixth edition, 1965; seventh edition (two volumes), 1972; and eighth edition (two volumes), 1978. *Tests in Print* was first published in 1961; the second edition is dated 1974, and a third edition is expected off the press by late 1983. *Intelligence Tests and Reviews* and *Vocational Tests and Reviews* were both published in 1975. *Personality Tests and Reviews* was published in 1970, with a second edition in 1975. The Gryphon Press in Highland Park, N.J., published all Buros Institute books through 1978. The publisher of current volumes is the University of Nebraska Press in Lincoln.

Acknowledgments

To all who have worked so hard to put this book into print, the editor offers sincere thanks.

If it were not for the progressive attitudes and constant positive reinforcement of all of my colleagues in the Department of Counseling of Gallaudet College's School of Education and Human Services, this project would still be on my shelf. Our secretarial staff of Dot Mallon and Karen Dickerson deserves badges of tolerance for typing predrafts, drafts, and post-drafts. Special mention must be made of four student contributors—Millie Brother, Margaret Stanton, L'Tanya Fish, and Scott Robinson—who made special efforts to ensure the accuracy of materials and to rewrite specific sections.

The brief summaries of reviews that appeared originally in the *Mental Measurements Yearbooks* or other publications of the Buros Institute of Mental Measurements are published with the permission of the Buros Institute of Mental Measurements of the University of Nebraska. All such material is protected by copyright. I wish to thank the Buros Institute for its cooperation and encouragement in this project.

Thanks are extended to members of Gallaudet College Press for their trust and hard work. I specifically appreciate the assistance of Jim Stentzel, who worked with me to ensure that the English language was not totally abused.

A personal note of thanks to Dr. Glenn Lloyd, Professor of Education at Lenoir Rhyne College and the editor of the *Journal of Rehabilitation of the Deaf.* He lit the spark for this text and, most importantly, had faith in my ability to complete it. I would also like to thank Dr. Ben Roth, my former professor and presently a practicing psychoanalyst in New York City. He taught me to respect tests and showed me the magical powers they hold in the hands of a competent practitioner.

A final word of special thanks to all contributors: Sleep well this night knowing that through your graduate program you not only gained a degree but made a valuable contribution to the lives of hearing-impaired people.

INTRODUCTION

GUIDELINES FOR SELECTING TESTS FOR HEARING-IMPAIRED CLIENTS

One of the questions most frequently asked of psychologists, counselors, and teachers who work with hearing-impaired people is, "What tests can I use with this population?" The most frequent answer is, "It depends."

A number of experts (Levine, 1981; Vernon, 1964; Watson, 1976) have attempted to assist professionals with a better answer than "It depends" by providing typical test batteries they have used or have seen used with hearing-impaired children, adolescents, and adults. Yet all of these experts would probably agree that the selection of appropriate tests for a hearing-impaired person does truly depend on two major factors: the nature of the client and the nature of the test.

Factors such as cause of hearing loss, age of onset, degree of loss, familial deafness, visual acuity, multiple handicapping conditions, mode of communication used in school and at home, speech production, and type of special education classes attended must be analyzed for each hearing-impaired individual before selecting test(s). There are a number of excellent references (Levine, 1981; Mindel & Vernon, 1971; Moores, 1978; Schlesinger & Meadow, 1972) that focus on each of these variables through discussions of the intellectual, social, and personality development of hearing-impaired people. An evaluator should study the ramifications of each variable in preparation for evaluating a hearing-impaired client.

This text focuses on the second major factor in selecting tests, that is, considerations of the nature of the test itself. There are four major questions that must be asked when choosing a test for a hearing-impaired person:

- Does the test consist of verbal test items or performance items?

- Do instructions for the test require verbal communication?

- Do any test items discriminate against an individual with an auditory impairment?

- Are hearing-impaired people included in the normative sample provided by the test developer?

Let us examine each of the questions to better understand the implications of the answers on the validity and/or reliability of test results for a hearing-impaired person.

The first criterion is the make-up of the test items themselves. Most tests can be categorized into two groups: verbal tests (reading and writing skills) and performance tests (manipulation of objects, tasks). Tests made up of verbal items are inappropriate for many hearing-impaired individuals, especially those individuals who became auditorally impaired before the normal development of language (approximately three years of age). Individuals in this category (prelingually deaf) usually have difficulty with English language syntax and vocabulary. Therefore, verbal test items may be misunderstood or misinterpreted by these people.

A good example of a test that brings this problem into focus is the Strong-Campbell Interest Inventory (Form T325). This verbal test is an excellent instrument to help most adolescents and adults discover occupational likes and dislikes and vocational attitude patterns. The authors purposely and properly designed the test so that it could be used with individuals who are reading at a sixth-grade level and above. This English comprehension level is appropriate for the majority of nonhandicapped adolescents who are juniors and seniors in high school. But this reading level is inappropriate for most prelingually hearing-impaired individuals, whose mean reading level (nationally) is estimated at a third- or fourth-grade level. Therefore, the validity of test results on the Strong-Campbell Inventory must be seriously questioned for some hearing-impaired individuals. The test results rarely reflect the vocational interests and attitudes of a hearing-impaired person; more often and more accurately, they reflect this person's English language deficiencies.

The second area of concern in test selection is the format of the instructions provided by the test developer. Does the test developer mandate the use of verbal instructions? Does the test developer present or permit alternate instruction procedures? These questions are important even if the test items themselves are performance tasks. If the individual being tested cannot fully comprehend the tasks required of him/her, the validity of the results must be questioned.

A good example of the problems that may occur from this criterion is found in the instructions provided for the performance subtests of the Wechsler Intelligence Tests (WAIS-R and WISC-R). Most experienced evaluators of hearing-impaired individuals would agree that the test items of all the subtests of the WAIS-R and WISC-R performance sections can be accomplished by a person with an auditory impairment. The nature of some of the instructions, however, creates a special problem. Wechsler clearly states in the manuals for both tests that the instructions should be given orally. Evaluators are not encouraged to alter instructions.

Most evaluators of hearing-impaired people have in fact altered the instructions of the WAIS-R and WISC-R using home-spun procedures of gestures, demonstration, sign language, and practice sheets. This decision may or may not be satisfactory, and its effectiveness usually depends on an evaluator's experience in attempting a variety of approaches with many hearing-impaired people.

There is no doubt that standardization of instruction procedures is lacking for many tests administered to hearing-impaired people, especially for tests designed with verbal instructions. Once again, validity of results becomes a major issue when this problem arises. The problem is more obvious when one compares test results of one hearing-impaired person instructed "by the book" with results of other hearing-impaired people given the same test but with a variety of instructional approaches.

The third criterion for test selection concerns the test items themselves. Do the test items relate directly or indirectly to an individual's ability to hear and function in a hearing world? Does any test item discriminate against an individual with a hearing impairment? This problem is most prevalent in intelligence, personality, and vocational interest test items.

A number of specific examples illustrate this problem. The Vineland Social Maturity Scale is a well-respected observational reporting scale used to assess social intelligence. Yet some of the behaviors included in the scale are inappropriate for some hearing-impaired people. Examples of behavior items for the Vineland Social Maturity Scale are "Talks, imitates sounds," "Talks in short sentences," "Reads on own initiative," and "Makes telephone calls."

The Wide Range Interest and Opinion Test—Revised is a vocational interest inventory using pictures to provoke personal likes and dislikes about job-related tasks. One set of three pictures shows an assembly line worker, a group of entertainers singing, and a telephone operator.

The Minnesota Multiphasic Personality Test is used for diagnosis of serious emotional disorders. Among the test statements are "When I am with people I am bothered by hearing very queer things," "My hearing is apparently as good as that of most people," and "I do not often notice my ears ringing or buzzing."

All of these examples come from well-designed and respected tests; and all of them discriminate unintentionally against auditory-disabled individuals. An evaluator must be cognizant of the fact that verbal communication is such a natural part of American society that we take this ability for granted even in test item construction.

The last criterion of test selection may be the most important and have the most far-reaching effect on hearing-impaired people: Does the test have normative data on hearing-impaired clients similar to your client? Add to this a more basic question: Did the test developer include handicapped people, and specifically hearing-impaired people, in the general normative sample?

This criterion is rarely met. Examples of tests that do have normative data on hearing-impaired clients are the WISC-R Adaptation by Ray; Stanford Achievement Test (Hearing-Impaired Edition); Geist Vocational Inventory: Deaf: Male Form; and the Hiskey-Nebraska Test of Learning Aptitude.

Normative data on hearing-impaired people become crucial in selective areas of psychological testing such as academic achievement, vocational aptitude, and work evaluation. For example, in evaluating the academic achievement of a hearing-impaired person, an evaluator can be in a tenuous situation if he/she compares the hearing-impaired client's results only with a national sampling of normal-hearing students. This may tell only half the story of a hearing-impaired person's true academic accomplishments and potential. The Stanford Achievement Test (Hearing-Impaired Edition) was designed to meet this need; it permits hearing-impaired clients' achievement scores to be compared with both hearing-impaired and normal-hearing peers.

The same problem exists with tests measuring vocational aptitude or work performance. Comparing a hearing-impaired person's test results with a normal-hearing population may sometimes be justified, but there are select and important situations where this is unwarranted or invalid.

If one were to eliminate from consideration all tests that do not have norms for hearing-impaired people—or tests that do not include hearing-impaired people within the general norm sample—we would in effect stop using standardized instruments to evaluate this group of people. For the pragmatists among us, this recommendation is unrealistic. What we can do is be very cautious about interpreting results of clients who do not mirror individuals for whom the test was designed.

This is a limited introduction to some of the "red flags" to consider when choosing tests for hearing-impaired people. As one sifts through the thousands of test instruments now available, an old adage becomes appropriate: "Consumer, beware!"

References

Levine, E. D. *The ecology of early deafness: Guides to fashioning environments and psychological assessments.* New York: Columbia University Press, 1981.

Mindel, E. D., & Vernon, M. *They grow in silence.* Silver Spring, Md.: National Association of the Deaf, 1971.

Moores, D. F. *Educating the deaf: Psychology, principles, and practices.* Boston: Houghton Mifflin, 1978.

Schlesinger, H. S., & Meadow, K. P. *Sound and sign.* Berkeley: University of California Press, 1972.

Vernon, M. A guide to psychological tests and testing procedures in the evaluation of deaf and hard-of-hearing children. *Journal of Speech and Hearing Disorders,* 1964, *29*(4), 414–423.

Watson, D. (Ed.). *Deaf evaluation and adjustment feasibility.* New York: New York University (Deafness Research and Training Center), 1976.

1

ACADEMIC ACHIEVEMENT TESTS

THE FULL-RANGE PICTURE VOCABULARY TEST

Author
R. B. Ammons and H. S. Ammons

Publisher
Psychological Test Specialists
Box 9229
Missoula, MT 59801

Price
$15.00 per set (cards, instructions, norms, and 25 record sheets)

Date of Edition
1948

General Purpose
The Full-Range Picture Vocabulary Test (FRPVT) was designed as a screening tool to give a rapid estimate of verbal comprehension for both children and adults.

Description
The FRPVT consists of 15 plates, each with four separate cartoon-like drawings. Approximately 80 words are used in each of the two parallel forms which cover the range of verbal abilities from early infancy to adulthood.

Administration
The FRPVT is administered individually. The individual is seated comfortably across a table from the examiner. The individual is asked to indicate by word or gesture which of the four pictures best illustrates the meaning of a given word. If the person does not seem to understand the procedure, further questions are asked using words other than those in the 226-item scale. The total time required for the test is 10 to 15 minutes.

Special Administration Procedures for Hearing-Impaired People
No special administration procedures for hearing-impaired people have been established.

Age Level

2 years and above

Reliability

Although the number of words involved in the FRPVT is relatively small, the reliability is quite adequate. This is not surprising in the area of vocabulary testing. For an adult sample, the authors report a reliability coefficient of .93 between Forms A and B. For the standardization groups, the median odd-even reliability for the various age levels is .81 and the coefficient for the full range of talent is .987.

Validity

Two correlations are provided to establish validity. One coefficient of .95 ($N=44$) is reported between the FRPVT and the Stanford-Binet vocabulary subtest. A coefficient of .86 was found between the FRPVT and the Wechsler-Bellevue Intelligence Scale.

Norms

Standardization was carried out on a population of 589 children and adults carefully controlled for age, sex, grade placement in school, and adult's or father's occupation. Norms based on the performance of this group appear on the back of each answer sheet. Separate norms have been set up for white farm children, Spanish-American children, Black children, and Black adults.

Norms for Hearing-Impaired People

None have been established.

Appropriateness for Hearing-Impaired People

This test requires simple yes/no responses. It can be administered to individuals who can communicate simply by pointing, nodding, or blinking. However, the individual must be able to receive the vocabulary word from the examiner in some way. This test seemingly could be administered through fingerspelling without upsetting the standard administration. Use of sign language should be discouraged because of lack of standardized signs and the fact that gestures may provide important clues to the appropriate answers.

Range of Scores

Raw scores are converted to percentiles and mental ages.

Interpretation

For children, the raw scores range from six through 69 with a raw score of six being equivalent to a mental age of 2.5 and a raw score of 69 being equivalent to a mental age of 16.5. For adults, the raw scores range from 52 to 84; a raw score of 52 is equivalent to a percentile score of one, and a raw score of 84 is equivalent to a percentile score of 99.

Summary of Buros Institute Publications

Discussed in the fourth and sixth editions of Buros's *Mental Measurements Yearbooks* (pp. 441-443 and pp. 806-807, respectively). The reviewers suggest the need for a concise, well-integrated test manual. They commend the usefulness of the FRPVT for individuals who have problems of limited comprehension of task directions, such as those in rehabilitation settings, and for people with communication difficulties or severe physical handicaps. They conclude that scores on the FRPVT provide a highly reliable and valid estimate of verbal intelligence for native-born, white, school-age children from urban and rural areas of the United States.

General References

Ammons, R. B., & Ammons, H. S. The Full-Range Vocabulary Test. *Abstract American Psychologist*, 1949, *4*, 267-268.

Ammons, R. B., Larson, W. L., & Shearn, C. R. The Full-Range Picture Vocabulary Test: Results for an adult population. *Journal of Clinical Psychology*, 1950, *14*, 150-155.

Joesting, J., & Joesting, R. Correlations of scores on Full-Range Picture Vocabulary Test: Three measures of creativity; SAT scores and age. *Pscyhological Report*, 1973, *33*, 981-982.

References Related to Hearing-Impaired People

Johnson, O. G. Testing the educational and psychological development of exceptional children. *Review of Educational Research*, 1968, *38*(1), 61-70.

GATES-MACGINITIE READING TESTS

Author
A. I. Gates and W. H. MacGinitie

Publisher
Riverside Publishing Company
1919 S. Highland Avenue
Lombard, IL 60148

Price
$10.74 per complete kit (package of 35 tests, teacher's guide, and scoring key)

Date of Edition
1978

General Purpose
The Gates-MacGinitie Reading Tests (GMRT) is a series of tests designed to determine a pupil's average reading level.

Description
The GMRT is based on age and grade levels as follows:

Primary A	Vocabulary & Comprehension (for grade 1)
Primary B	Vocabulary & Comprehension (grade 2)
Primary C	Vocabulary & Comprehension (grade 3)
Primary CS	Speed & Accuracy (grades 2 & 3)
Survey D	Speed, Vocabulary, & Comprehension (grades 4 to 6)
Survey E	Speed, Vocabulary, & Comprehension (grades 7 to 9)
Survey F	Speed, Vocabulary, & Comprehension (grades 10 to 12)

Administration
The GMRT may be administered individually or to a group. Directions suggest 20 to 30 minutes for the vocabulary subtests and approximately 30 minutes for comprehension subtests. The speed subtests require 10 minutes for grades three, four, and five, and 7 minutes for grades six and above. Sample tests may be used. Each part of the test should be given in the order prescribed by the author. Answer sheets are provided.

Special Administration Procedures for Hearing-Impaired People
No special administration procedures for hearing-impaired people have been established. Instructions should be given through appropriate means of communication (sign language, gestures, etc.), with ample time for sample items.

Age Level
Kindergarten through grade 12

Reliability
Reliability coefficients were derived by using alternate form and split-half reliabilities. Alternate form reliability coefficients ranged from .67 to .89. Split-half reliability coefficients ranged from .88 to .96.

Validity
Concurrent validity coefficients for form Primary C at grade three and Survey D at grade five were obtained with four other standardized reading tests. Median validity coefficients were .84 for Primary C vocabulary, .79 for Primary C comprehension, .78 for Survey D vocabulary, and .80 for Survey D comprehension.

Norms
The 1964-65 norms for the GMRT were developed by administering the tests to a nationwide sample of approximately 40,000 students in 37 communities. The communities were selected on the basis of size, geographical location, educational level, and family income. Within each community testing was carried out in one or more schools judged by the school officials to be representative of the community.

Norms for Hearing-Impaired People
None have been established.

Appropriateness for Hearing-Impaired People
The vocabulary sections of Primary A, B, and C subtests appear to be appropriate for use with hearing-impaired children. The comprehension sections of Primary A, B, and C subtests; Primary CS; and Surveys D, E, and F may not be appropriate because they require advanced reading levels.

8 / Assessment of Hearing-Impaired People

Range of Scores

Raw scores are converted to *T*-scores with a mean of 50 and a standard deviation of 10.

Interpretation

The GMRT determines a student's average reading level and provides information appropriate for decisions of educational placement and remedial services.

Summary of Buros Institute Publications

Discussed in the seventh edition of Buros's *Mental Measurements Yearbook* (Vol. 2, pp. 1080–1085). The reviewers feel that the present series of tests is a marked improvement over previous editions. The manuals are complete and well-organized. The norming groups are adequate. The directions for administrators are clear. The GMRT compares favorably with other general reading tests, providing valuable data on achievement in comprehension, vocabulary, and speed.

General References

Davis, W. Q. *A study of test score compatability among five widely used reading survey-tests.* Unpublished doctoral dissertation, Southern Illinois University, 1968.

Gates, A. I. *The improvement of reading: A program of diagnostic and remedial methods* (3rd ed.). New York: Macmillan, 1947.

Thorndike, R. L. *The concepts of over-and-underachievement.* New York: Teachers College Press, 1963.

References Related to Hearing-Impaired People

Furth, H. G. A comparison of reading test norms of deaf and hearing children. *Americans Annals of the Deaf,* 1966, *111*(2), 461–462.

Giangreco, C. J. The Hiskey-Nebraska Test of Learning Aptitude (Revised) compared to several achievement tests. *American Annals of the Deaf,* 1966, *111*(4), 566–577.

KEY MATH
DIAGNOSTIC ARITHMETIC TEST

Author

A. Connolly, W. Nachtman, and M. Pritchett

Publisher

American Guidance Service, Inc.
Publishers Building
Circle Pines, MN 55014

Price

$35.00 per kit (easel, 25 booklets, and manual)

Date of Edition

1976

General Purpose

Key Math is designed to provide a diagnostic assessment of skills in mathematics.

Description

In order to spur motivation, the test material is colorful and arranged in an easel kit for quick and efficient administration. It is divided into 14 subtests organized into three major areas—*content* (numeration, fractions, geometry, and symbols); *operations* (addition, subtraction, multiplication, division, mental computation, and numerical reasoning); and *applications* (word problems, missing elements, money, measurement, and time).

Administration

Key Math is an individually administered power test, not a speed test. Administration time will vary according to the strength and work habits of the children. Most items require the students to respond verbally to open-ended items which are presented orally by the examiner. The goal is to test the child on items within his/her critical range of knowledge. This range extends from a basal level established by three consecutive correct responses to a ceiling level identified by three consecutive errors. The total time required is 30 minutes.

Special Administration Procedures for Hearing-Impaired People

No special administration procedures for hearing-impaired people have been established.

Age Level

Kindergarten through grade 7

Reliability

Reliable coefficients ranged from .94 to .97. These correlations were derived from a split-half analysis of the norming population's performance on Key Math by grade level.

Validity

A correlation coefficient of .59 was found between the performance on Key Math and the measured intelligence of 45 educable, mentally retarded adolescents. A correlation coefficient of .69 was found with Key Math and the arithmetic portions of the Iowa Test of Basic Skills. A coefficient of .38 was found with the full-scale Iowa Arithmetic Test score.

Norms

The Key Math norming consisted of 1,222 children drawn from grades K through 7. The sample included 42 schools in 21 school districts from eight states. The schools were randomly selected and the population was formed by randomly selecting six pupils at each grade level. The sample of schools contained a wide range of geographic and racial representation from urban, suburban, and rural settings.

Norms for Hearing-Impaired People

None have been established.

Appropriateness for Hearing-Impaired People

Caution must be used in administering this test to a hearing-impaired person. Because many items require oral instructions and verbal responses, communication between examiner and child is vital. Written instructions and written responses should not be used.

Range of Scores

Raw scores are converted to grade equivalents. A norm table of grade equivalent scores is presented in the manual.

Interpretation

Key Math delineates in considerable detail the mathematical deficit areas of the child. This enables the teacher to use this test diagnostically and to plan precise remedial programs.

Summary of Buros Institute Publications

Discussed in the eighth edition of Buros's *Mental Measurements Yearbook* (Vol. 1, pp. 451–452). According to the reviewers, Key Math is standardized on a sufficient sample of individuals and has demonstrated satisfactory reliability and validity. The reviewers recommend at least five trial administrations before using it diagnostically. Key Math should become a standard part of the test battery of everyone concerned with evaluating and treating learning-disabled children.

General References

Cawley, J. R., Goodstein, H. A., Fitzmaurice, A. M., Lepore, A., Sedlak, R., & Althaus, V. *Mathematics activities for teaching the handicapped.* Storrs: University of Connecticut, 1974.

Kramer, K. *The teaching of elementary school mathematics.* Boston: Allyn and Bacon, 1966.

Lowell, K. *The growth of basic mathematical and scientific concepts in children.* London: University of London, 1961.

Tinney, F. A. A comparison of the Key Math Diagnostic Arithmetic Test and the California Arithmetic Test used with learning disabled students. *Journal of Learning Disabilities,* 1975, 8, 57–59.

References Related to Hearing-Impaired People

None available

METROPOLITAN ACHIEVEMENT TESTS SERIES

Author
I. H. Balow, R. Farr, T. Hogan, and G. A. Prescott

Publisher
The Psychological Corporation
757 Third Avenue
New York, NY 10017

Price
$3.50 to $4.25 per manual for each battery level
$5.00 per specimen set of each battery level

Date of Edition
1979

General Purpose
The Metropolitan Achievement Tests (MAT) Series is a dependable battery designed to provide information on pupil achievement in several important skill and content areas of a general school curriculum.

Description
The MAT consists of eight battery levels measuring performance from the beginning of kindergarten through grade 12. The eight battery levels are: *Preprimer, Primer, Primary 1, Primary 2, Elementary, Intermediate, Advanced 1,* and *Advanced 2*. Each battery level consists of different combinations of subtests which may include subtests of reading comprehension, mathematics, language, social studies, and science.

Administration
The MAT is designed for teacher administration in a group setting. At all levels, the directions for administration are exceptionally thorough and clear. The inclusion of a separate practice sheet for the primer level should serve to prepare students for testing. Administration of the complete battery may extend over a few days.

Special Administration Procedures for Hearing-Impaired People
No specific guidelines are provided for administering the MAT to hearing-impaired students.

Age Level
Grades K.0 to 12.9

Reliability
Reliability estimates are based on measures of internal consistency. The correlations are typically .90 or higher for each of the various subtests at each grade level.

Validity
National content validation was conducted using extensive analyses of textbooks, syllabi, state guidelines, and other curricular sources. Detailed instructional objectives, used as one guide for selecting items, were obtained from more than 10,000 teachers nationwide.

Norms
A distinctive aspect of the MAT standardization program is that initial testing was conducted in both the fall and spring, eliminating the need to interpolate norms for different midyear grade levels. The MAT normative sample was based on voluntary participation of a national sample of schools and involved the testing of more than 550,000 pupils. Standardization samples were selected to represent a national school population with respect to public versus nonpublic school affiliation, geographic region, socioeconomic status, and ethnic background.

Norms for Hearing-Impaired People
None have been established.

Appropriateness for Hearing-Impaired People
The major weakness of the MAT compared with other achievement tests such as the Stanford Achievement Test (Hearing-Impaired Edition) is the lack of appropriate norms for hearing-impaired children. This is vital information, since the goal of all achievement tests is to compare a child's results with his/her peers.

Range of Scores

Raw scores are converted to scaled scores (continuous through all levels), percentile ranks, stanines, normal curve equivalents, and grade equivalents. The manual clearly describes the limitation of grade equivalents and urges that they be used only for the interpretation of averages and not for the interpretation of individual scores.

Interpretation

Test results can be used for purposes of educational and vocational placement, remedial academic services, and prescriptive educational planning.

Summary of Buros Institute Publications

An earlier edition of the MAT was reviewed in the eighth edition of Buros's *Mental Measurements Yearbook* (Vol. 1, pp. 63-71). According to the reviewers, the 1970 edition of the MAT measures important skill and knowledge outcomes. The directions for administering the test at all levels are clear. The format is attractive throughout. The MAT provides a high quality interpretive aid for the user. The major criticism of the 1970 edition was the age of the items, which were based on curriculum material more than ten years old. Although the 1979 edition of the MAT has not been reviewed in Buros's *Mental Measurements Yearbooks*, it would appear that the updating of items would answer the major criticism of the 1970 edition.

General References

Crockett, B. K., Rardin, M. W., & Pasewark, R. A. Relationship of WPPSI and subsequent Metropolitan Achievement Test scores in Head-Start children. *Psychology in the Schools,* 1976, *13*(1), 19-20.

Davenport, B. M. A comparison of the Peabody Individual Achievement Test, the Metropolitan Achievement Test, and the Otis-Lennon Mental Ability Test. *Psychology in the Schools,* 1976 *13*(3), 291-297.

Yoshida, R. K. Out-of-level testing of special education students with a standardized achievement battery. *Journal of Educational Measurements,* 1976, *13*(3), 215-221.

References Related to Hearing-Impaired People

Giangreco, C. J. The Hiskey-Nebraska Test of Learning Aptitude (Revised) compared to several achievement tests. *American Annals of the Deaf,* 1966, *111*(4), 566-577.

Hess, D. W. Evaluation of the young deaf adult. *Journal of Rehabilitation of the Deaf,* 1969, *3*(2), 6-21.

PEABODY PICTURE VOCABULARY TEST

Author
L. N. Dunn

Publisher
American Guidance Service, Inc.
Publishers Building
Circle Pines, MN 55014

Price
$10.00 (examiner's kit of picture booklet, 25 individual records for Forms A and B, and manual)

Date of Edition
1965

General Purpose
The Peabody Picture Vocabulary Test (PPVT) is designed to provide a rapid measurement of "use" vocabulary and is especially applicable to persons unable to vocalize well. It is widely used to evaluate a child's comprehension of words as well as to provide an estimate of the child's verbal intelligence.

Description
The PPVT consists of a booklet with three practice and 150 test plates, each containing four numbered pictures. The same booklet is used for Forms A and B; the forms differ only in the stimulus word/correct picture response for each of the 150 items.

Administration
The PPVT is designed to be administered individually. As each plate is presented, the examiner provides a stimulus word orally; the child responds by pointing to or in some other way designating the picture on the plate that best illustrates the meaning of the stimulus word. Each individual is given only the plates appropriate to his/her own performance level. The test is untimed and usually is completed in less than 15 minutes.

Special Administration Procedures for Hearing-Impaired People
No special administration procedures for hearing-impaired people have been established. Stimulus words may be pronounced aloud more than once by the examiner.

Age Level
29 months to 18 years

Reliability
Alternate form reliability coefficients for the PPVT were obtained by calculating Pearson product-moment correlations on the raw scores of the standardization sample for Forms A and B at each level. For the different age levels, the coefficients ranged from a low of .67 at the six-year level to a high of .84 at the 17–18-year levels, with a median of .77. The standard error of measurement for IQ scores ranged from 6.00 to 8.61, the median being 7.20. Reliability coefficients within the same range were subsequently obtained with several mentally retarded and physically handicapped groups. The coefficients ranged from .54 to .97.

Validity
Validity was originally established in terms of age differentiation. Since publication, the PPVT has been used in a number of studies with normal, mentally retarded, emotionally disturbed, and physically handicapped children. These studies have yielded validity coefficients in the .60s with relatively homogeneous age groups. There is also some evidence of moderate concurrent and predictive validity with academic achievement tests. A limitation of this test for certain testing purposes is that culturally disadvantaged children tend to perform more poorly on it than on other intelligence tests.

Norms
A total of 4,012 children were administered both Forms A and B of the final battery by four examiners between April and June 1958. The alternate forms were counterbalanced by order of presentation. The sample was comprised of white children residing in and around Nashville, Tennessee. According to the authors, certain precautions were taken to provide norms which should be useful throughout the United States.

Norms for Hearing-Impaired People

None have been established.

Appropriateness for Hearing-Impaired People

The PPVT manual states that the examiner must not spell, define, or even show the word to the examinee, but nothing is said about the use of sign language. Because specific signs have not been standardized, comparison of results from deaf children would not be valid. Therefore, unless a child can fully understand the vocabulary words through the speech of the examiner, this test would appear inappropriate for most hearing-impaired children.

Range of Scores

Raw scores can be converted to three types of derived scores: percentiles, mental ages, and intelligence quotients. Intelligence quotient scores range from 55 to 145 with a mean of 100 and a standard deviation of 15.

Interpretation

Intelligence Quotients	Percent	Classification
125 and above	5	very rapid learners
110 to 124	20	rapid learners
90 to 109	50	average learners
75 to 89	20	slow learners
below 75	5	very slow learners

Summary of Buros Institute Publications

As discussed in the sixth edition of Buros's *Mental Measurements Yearbook* (pp. 820-823), the PPVT is probably the best test of its kind. It is a highly usable test of moderate reliability and largely established validity.

General References

Allen, R. M., Haupt, T. D., & Jones, R. W. A suggested use and non-use of the Peabody Picture Vocabulary Test with the retarded child. *Psychology Report*, 1964, *15*, 421-422.

Mueller, M. Effects of illustration size on PPVT test performance of visually limited children. *Exceptional Children*, 1962, *29*, 124-128.

Norris, R. C., Hottel, J. V., & Brooks, S. Comparability of Peabody Picture Vocabulary Test scores under group and individual administration. *Journal of Educational Psychology*, 1960, *51*, 87-91.

References Related to Hearing-Impaired People

Corwin, B. J. *The influence of culture and language on performance on individual ability tests*. Unpublished study, San Fernando Valley State College (Division of Education), 1962.

Hedger, M. F. An analysis of three picture vocabulary tests for use with the deaf. In J. Rosenstein & W. H. MacGinitie (Eds.), *Research on the psycholinguistic behavior of deaf children* (Rev. ed.). Washington, D.C.: Council for Exceptional Children, 1964. (Monograph)

STANFORD ACHIEVEMENT TEST
Special Edition for Hearing-Impaired Students

Author
R. Madden, E. Gardner, H. Rudman, B. Karlsen, and J. Merwin (Stanford Achievement Test)

Office of Demographic Studies, Gallaudet College (Hearing-Impaired Edition)

Publisher
Harcourt Brace Jovanovich, Inc.
727 Third Avenue
New York, NY 10017

Price
$16.00 (sample test with manual and key)

Date of Edition
1973

General Purpose
The Stanford Achievement Test, Special Edition for Hearing-Impaired Students (SAT-HI) is an adaptation of the 1973 edition of the Stanford Achievement Test (SAT). It was adapted by the Office of Demographic Studies (now the Center for Assessment and Demographic Studies) at Gallaudet College, to which any inquiries should be directed. The purpose of the special edition is to measure the academic achievement of hearing-impaired students. A revision of the SAT was completed in 1982. A revision of the SAT-HI is expected by late 1983 or early 1984.

Description
The SAT-HI is a full-range achievement test. It consists of six different levels or batteries: primary level 1, level 2, level 3, level 4, level 5, and advanced level. There are four core subject areas: vocabulary, reading comprehension, mathematics concepts, and mathematics computation. Recommended practice tests are available for all test levels.

Administration
The SAT-HI is designed to be administered in a group setting, specifically the children's classroom. Practice tests are provided for each level and subtest. The direction manuals for each of the levels provide a proposed schedule for administering the test batteries. When administering test items, the wording in the manual must be followed exactly; however, when explaining directions, it is permissible to expand, elaborate, explain, and demonstrate. The method of communication normally used in the classroom should also be used during the testing. The entire test should be completed within one week.

Special Administration Procedures for Hearing-Impaired People
The SAT-HI was designed for hearing-impaired students. The above administration procedures should be followed. Two special features of the SAT-HI are practice tests for subtests and procedures for choosing appropriate reading levels for hearing-impaired children.

Age Level
8 to 21 years

Reliability
A reliability coefficient of .83 was derived by averaging the reliability coefficients for all subtests in the different test batteries. The reliability coefficients were derived from correlations by test-retest methods used with a standardized group. The standard error of measurement (SEM) is 3.0. This was derived from the average of all the SEMs of the subtests of the different test batteries. Refer to Jensema (1978) for complete reliability and SEM tables.

Validity
No studies of validity specifically for the SAT-HI are reported. Because test items of the SAT-HI and SAT are exactly the same, the authors assume that content validity will not vary between tests.

Norms

The SAT was standardized on a national sample of 275,000 school children in grades one to nine. The sample was chosen in accordance with the 1970 U.S. Census and stratified proportionally according to ethnic minorities, geographic regions, parental incomes, educational levels of communities, and major schools characteristics.

Norms for Hearing-Impaired People

Norms are based on the performance of a carefully selected random sample of 6,873 hearing-impaired students in 119 special education programs throughout the United States. This sample included gifted as well as academically slow, hearing-impaired children. Age-based percentile norms for hearing-impaired students were developed from this sample.

Appropriateness for Hearing-Impaired People

The SAT-HI was designed specifically for hearing-impaired children and adolescents and therefore is appropriate and recommended.

Range of Scores

Raw scores are converted into grade equivalent scores, scaled scores, and percentiles. The grade equivalent scores range from K.1 through 12.9, while the scaled scores range from 42 through 300. The child's results on the SAT-HI may be compared to hearing as well as hearing-impaired peers nationally.

Interpretation

The results may be used as one of multiple measures of academic achievement for the purposes of school and grade placement, remedial academic services, and prescriptive educational planning.

Summary of Buros Institute Publications

The SAT-HI is not reviewed in Buros's *Mental Measurements Yearbooks*. The 1973 edition of the Stanford Achievement Test is reviewed in the eighth edition of the yearbook (Vol. 1, pp. 96-107). The reviewers feel that the SAT is an excellent achievement test. It is the best available, ongoing assessment of basic skills from elementary through junior high school levels.

General References

Not relevant

References Related to Hearing-Impaired People

Brill, R. G. The superior IQ's of deaf children of deaf parents. *Journal of Rehabilitation of the Deaf,* 1970, *4*(2), 45-53.

Jensema, C. A. A comment on measurement error in achievement tests for the hearing impaired. *American Annals of the Deaf,* 1978, *123*(4), 496-499.

Karchmer, M. A., Milone, M. N., & Wolk, S. Educational significance of hearing loss at three levels of severity. *American Annals of the Deaf,* 1979, *124*(2), 97-109.

Trybus, R. J., & Jensema, C. The development, use, and interpretation of the 1973 Stanford Achievement Test, Special Edition for Hearing-Impaired Students. In *Report of Proceedings of the Forty-seventh Meeting of the Convention of American Instructors of the Deaf.* Washington, D.C.: Government Printing Office, 1976.

Trybus, R. J., and Karchmer, M. A. School achievement scores of hearing-impaired children: National data on achievement status and growth patterns. *American Annals of the Deaf,* 1977, *122*(2), 62-69.

Verbal Language Development Scale

Author
M. J. Mecham

Publisher
American Guidance Service, Inc.
Publishers Building
Circle Pines, MN 55014

Price
$2.90 (package of 25 tests)
$1.20 (manual)

Date of Edition
1971

General Purpose
The Verbal Language Development Scale (VLDS) is an extension of the communication portion of the Vineland Social Maturity Scale. Like the Vineland Scale, it is designed as an indirect method of assessing a child's daily-life communicative skills when direct testing methods prove unreliable because of severe physical or emotional problems.

Description
The VLDS consists of 50 items that the examiner asks of an informant (an individual who has a close relationship with the client). Interviewing a parent or teacher is preferable. The scale is divided into nine age-levels. The questions are based on a child's listening, speaking, writing, and reading abilities at each of the age levels.

Administration
The VLDS is designed to be administered individually. Using the informant-interview method of administration, the examiner elicits information regarding the client's behavior. Each item contains a definition of the behavior being sought. The examiner begins the questioning with those items one year below the chronological age of the client. When eight consecutive positive scores are received, the examiner can proceed up the scale; if not, he or she moves down the scale until there are eight positive responses. The test is completed either when all 50 items have been answered or when eight consecutive negative scores have been tallied. The total time required ranges from 30 to 45 minutes.

Special Administration Procedures for Hearing-Impaired People
No special administration procedures for hearing-impaired people have been established.

Age Level
Birth to 15 years

Reliability
Test-retest estimates of reliability were derived from 15 children of the original norm group. A coefficient of .96 was found using the rank-difference procedure. A correlation of .96 was derived from a study of 28 mentally retarded children using an alternate form reliability procedure. Comparisons of scores from a direct-test form and an informant-interview form provided reliability coefficients ranging from .72 to .97.

Validity
A one-way-analysis-of-variance by ranks showed an *H*-score of 120.8 which is significant at the .001 level. Using a sample of 92 mentally retarded children, a comparison of scores from the VLDS and the Stanford-Binet Form L yielded coefficients of .72, .79 (for educationally trainable children), and .93 (for severely mentally retarded children). A sample of 40 deaf children was tested to ensure that the VLDS measured language skills and not intelligence. The difference between language and intelligence scores was significant at the .01 level.

Norms
Scores were derived from an original sample of 120 normal-speaking white children representative of central Utah in respect to age, sex, socioeconomic background, and residence. Additional information was gathered from a second sample of 117 children from mid-northern Utah. Criteria for selection were the same for this group.

Norms for Hearing-Impaired People

None have been established.

Appropriateness for Hearing-Impaired People

The VLDS appears to be inappropriate for most hearing-impaired children. Although the informant-interview technique is advantageous for evaluators unable to communicate with hearing-impaired people, the test items discriminate against auditory impairments. Comparison of results with normal-hearing children is invalid. Unless local norms are developed for hearing-impaired students, the test should not be used.

Range of Scores

The VLDS results are presented in raw scores ranging from 1.0 to 50.0. A positive score (earning one credit point) is given if the informant indicates that the child routinely exhibits the behavior in question. One-half credit point is given if the behavior is in a transitional or emergent state. The total score is the sum of all full and half points.

Interpretation

Using the total raw score, a language-age equivalent can be found by referring to Table 2 of the manual.

Summary of Buros Institute Publications

Discussed in the seventh edition of Buros's *Mental Measurements Yearbook* (Vol. 2, pp. 1368–1370). The reviewers recommend that the test be used with appropriate caution, as a screening device, not a diagnostic instrument, to assess a child's expressive and receptive language ability.

General References

Mecham, M. J., & Case, J. L. Comparison of two approaches to the assessment of verbal language development of mentally retarded children: A review. *Digest of the Mentally Retarded*, 1968, *5*, 29–32.

Wilhaus, W. G. Adequacy and usefulness of an objective language scale when administered to elementary school children. *Journal of Educational Research*, 1960, *54*, 30–33.

References Related to Hearing-Impaired People

Bown, J. C., & Mecham, M. J. The assessment of verbal language development in deaf children. *Volta Review*, 1961, *63*, 228–230.

WIDE RANGE ACHIEVEMENT TEST

Author
J. F. Jastak, S. Bijou, and S. R. Jastak

Publisher
Jastak Associates, Inc.
1526 Gilpin Avenue
Wilmington, DE 19806

Price
$9.75 (package of 50 test booklets)
$13.65 (manual)

Date of Edition
1978

General Purpose
The Wide Range Achievement Test (WRAT), first standardized in 1936, has undergone four revisions. The test is designed to measure levels of competence in basic school subjects.

Description
The WRAT has two levels (see Age Level) based on the difficulty of material. Each level consists of three subtests: *reading* (recognizing and naming letters and pronouncing words out of context); *spelling* (copying marks resembling letters, writing the name, and writing single words to dictation); and *arithmetic* (counting, reading number symbols, solving oral problems, and performing written computations).

Administration
The WRAT is basically an individually administered test with provision for group administration of some subtests. The timing for each of the subtests varies. An oral section is provided for each of the subtests; it is used when the written method is inappropriate (e.g., because of blindness). The three subtests may be given in any convenient order. The total time required ranges from 45 to 60 minutes.

Special Administration Procedures for Hearing-Impaired People
No special administration procedures for hearing-impaired people have been established. There are special considerations for administering some subtests to blind people.

Age Level
Level I: 5 years, 0 months to 11 years, 11 months
Level II: 12 years, 0 months to adulthood

Reliability
According to the author, the WRAT satisfies statistical conditions of reliability adequately. From numerous studies of a variety of populations, the authors report reliability correlation coefficients ranging from .92 to .98 for the reading and spelling subtests and from .85 to .92 for the arithmetic subtest.

Validity
The validity of the WRAT was determined through several different methods: (1) correlation of scores with other achievement tests; (2) correlation of test results with teacher ratings; (3) correlation of scores with measures of intelligence or mental ability; and (4) factor analysis of a large number of abilities to determine the factor loadings inherent in each subtest. Results of numerous research studies on the validity of the WRAT are provided in the manual. Validity coefficients vary widely depending on the criteria used.

Norms
The revised 1978 WRAT was administered to more than 15,200 people (children and adults) in seven states. No attempt was made to obtain a representative national sampling. The sample was in no way restricted to any economic, intellectual, or racial groups. Norm tables are provided by age and sex. Each age grouping has equal representation of males and females.

Norms for Hearing-Impaired People
None have been established.

Appropriateness for Hearing-Impaired People

For the most part, the 1978 WRAT is inappropriate for many hearing-impaired persons. Most subtests are administered orally and therefore discriminate against hearing-impaired people who rely on sign language or other visual cues. In addition, the lack of hearing-impaired norms limits comparison and interpretation of individual results.

Range of Scores

Raw scores are converted to grade ratings, percentiles, and standard scores. A standard score may also be converted to a *T*-score, stanine, or scaled score for research purposes.

Interpretation

The numerical results of the WRAT serve a variety of purposes: determination of instructional levels for school children, determination of degrees of literacy and arithmetic proficiency of mentally retarded persons, selection or promotion of personnel at various occupational levels, selection of students for specialized technical and professional schools, and comparison between school achievement and other abilities in all individuals, especially those who are disturbed or maladjusted.

Summary of Buros Institute Publications

Earlier editions of the WRAT are discussed in the seventh edition of Buros's *Mental Measurements Yearbook* (Vol. 1, pp. 65–68). The reviewers are highly critical of its validity and reliability studies. They also criticize administration procedures for being complex and confusing.

General References

Ayres, A. Deficits in sensory integration in educationally handicapped children. *Journal of Learning Disabilities*, 1969, *2*, 654–656.

Washington, E. D., & Teska, J. A. Relations between the Wide Range Achievement Test, the California Achievement Test, the Stanford-Binet, and the Illinois Test of Psycholinguistic Abilities. *Psychological Reports*, 1970, *26*, 291–294.

References Related to Hearing-Impaired People

Bonham, S. J., Jr. *Predicting achievement for deaf children* (Dayton City School District). Columbus: Ohio State Department of Education, 1963.

WOODCOCK READING MASTERY TESTS

Author
R. W. Woodcock

Publisher
American Guidance Service, Inc.
Publishers Building
Circle Pines, MN 55014

Price
Form A: $29.50 (complete test kit)
Form B: $29.50 (complete test kit)

Date of Edition
1973

General Purpose

The Woodcock Reading Mastery Tests (WRMT) is a carefully constructed series of individual reading tasks. The fundamental objective of this battery of tests is to provide precise measures of reading ability for clinical or research purposes.

Description

The test booklet is a sturdy easel-type ring-binder which is placed between the test-taker and the administrator. The booklet contains five subtests: *letter identification, word identification, word attack, word comprehension*, and *passage comprehension*. The test is available in two alternate forms, A and B.

Administration

The WRMT is designed to be administered individually. The test questions are open-ended. The examinee begins the letter identification subtest and word attack subtest with the first items. In the remaining subtests the examiner estimates the examinee's reading level; a suggested starting point for that level is provided in the directions. The starting point, hopefully, will closely correspond with the basal level (five consecutive right answers); the examinee continues the test until the ceiling level (unable to answer five consecutive questions) or the last question is reached. The total time required ranges from 20 to 40 minutes.

Special Administration Procedures for Hearing-Impaired People

No special administration procedures for hearing-impaired people have been established.

Age Level

Kindergarten through grade 12

Reliability

Split-half reliabilities for the five subtests were in the .90 to .99 range. Test-retest reliability coefficients ranged from .16 to .94 with a median coefficient of .84.

Validity

Evidence related to validity is provided using a number of methods including a multitrait, multimethod matrix analysis. Based on 103 individuals, this method of analysis yielded validity coefficients ranging from .84 to .94.

Norms

Norms are based on the test results of approximately 5,000 pupils from kindergarten through grade 12. The norming sample was a stratified random sample of pupils enrolled in regular classrooms. Communities throughout the United States were selected to ensure wide socioeconomic and geographic representation.

Norms for Hearing-Impaired People

No norms have been established.

Appropriateness for Hearing-Impaired People

The WRMT is an inappropriate measure of reading skills for many hearing-impaired children. Two subtests require oral responses for phonetic analysis; two subtests consist of very sophisticated language. The other subtest, letter identification, is an effective measure of reading ability only for very young children. The lack of hearing-impaired norms limits comparison and interpretation of results.

Range of Scores

Raw scores are converted into mastery scores which are then used to obtain standard scores. The standard scores range from 27 to 73 with a mean of 50 and a standard deviation of 10. Percentiles and stanine scores are also provided.

Interpretation

Results of the WRMT are most often used for educational placement and identification of specific remedial services that may be needed.

Summary of Buros Institute Publications

Discussed in the eighth edition of Buros's *Mental Measurements Yearbook* (Vol. 2, pp. 1303-1311). The reviewers are highly critical of reported validity studies. The test makes claims to innovation and technical quality not supported by data. Although the test is not recommended for general use, it may be a valuable tool in the hands of an experienced reading diagnostician.

General References

Bannatyne, A. Review of the Woodcock Reading Tests. *Journal of Learning Disabilities*, 1974, *7*, 398-399.

Allington, R. Review of the Woodcock Reading Tests. *Journal of Reading*, 1976, *2*, 162-163.

Houck, C., & Harris, L. Review of the Woodcock Reading Mastery Tests. *Journal of School Psychology*, 1976, *1*, 77-79.

References Related to Hearing-Impaired People

None available

2 COMMUNICATION TESTS

DENVER SCALE OF COMMUNICATION FUNCTION

Author

J. Alpiner, W. Chevrette, G. Glascoe, M. Metz, and B. Olsen

Publisher

Not commercially available. Permission to copy the scale may be obtained by writing: Dr. Jerome G. Alpiner, Department of Communication Disorders, University of Mississippi, University, MS 38677

Price

Not provided

Date of Edition

Copyright 1974; printed in J. G. Alpiner (Ed.), *The Handbook of Adult Rehabilitative Audiology*. Baltimore: William & Wilkins, 1978.

General Purpose

The Denver Scale of Communication Function (DSCF) is designed to help the clinician assess communication attitudes of adults with acquired hearing loss. The purpose of the scale is to focus attention on improving the client's communication.

Description

The DSCF consists of four sample questions followed by 25 questions. The client judges his or her own communication functioning in four categories: family, self, social-vocational, and general communication experience. Answers are designed in a seven-point scale ranging from "strongly agree" to "strongly disagree."

Administration

The DSCF is designed to be administered individually. The examiner records client's biographical data, pure tone and discrimination scores, and hearing aid information. The scale is reviewed with the client; then the client answers the 25 questions independently. To encourage first-impression responses, a 15-minute time limit is set for completion of the entire scale.

Special Administration Procedures for Hearing-Impaired People

The scale was designed to be administered to hearing-impaired adults with acquired hearing loss.

Age Level

Adults

Reliability

In a reliability study by McNeil (1975), test-retest reliability on a sample of eight people yielded a correlation coefficient of .729. Using the split-half measure of reliability, more than one-third of the total (nine) was found unreliable.

Validity

Concurrent validity coefficients ranged from .415 to .953. A simple, one-way analysis of variance was computed. None of the results were significant at the .01 level of confidence.

Norms

None have been established.

Norms for Hearing-Impaired People

No norms have been established; however, Schow and Nerbonne at Idaho State University are currently compiling data.

Appropriateness for Hearing-Impaired People

The DSCF, according to Alpiner, is appropriate for adults with an acquired hearing loss.

Range of Scores

A categorical range from strong agreement to strong disagreement is obtained.

Interpretation

Interpretation of the DSCF depends heavily on the skill and experience of the audiologist. As an audiological assessment tool, the scale is helpful in planning remediation of communication ability.

Summary of Buros Institute Publications

Not reviewed in Buros's *Mental Measurements Yearbooks*

General References

None available

References Related to Hearing-Impaired People

Alpiner, J. G. (Ed.). *The handbook of adult rehabilitative audiology*. Baltimore: William & Wilkins, 1978.

McNeil, M.R. *A study of the reliability of the Denver Scale of Communication Function*. Unpublished study, University of Denver, 1975.

ILLINOIS TEST OF PSYCHOLINGUISTIC ABILITIES (REVISED)

Author
S. A. Kirk, J. J. McCarthy, and W. D. Kirk

Publisher
University of Illinois Press
Urbana, IL 61801

Price
$105.00 (complete kit)

Date of Edition
1968

General Purpose
The Illinois Test of Psycholinguistic Abilities (ITPA) is designed as a test of language, perception, and short-term memory abilities.

Description
The ITPA is an aptitude test designed to assess psycholinguistic abilities in the English language. The ITPA consists of ten subtests: *auditory reception, visual reception, auditory association, visual association, verbal expression, manual expression, grammatic closure, visual closure, auditory sequential memory,* and *visual sequential memory.* There are also two supplementary subtests: *auditory closure* and *sound blending.*

Administration
The ITPA is designed to be administered individually. Specific instructions must be given to the children in a clear and understandable manner. There are two examples for each subtest to be used with the directions. The examiner needs practice in managing the items so that the test can be given in one session for most children and preferably in less than one hour.

Special Administration Procedures for Hearing-Impaired People
No special administration procedures for hearing-impaired people have been established.

Age Level
2- to 10-year-old children from English-speaking environments

Reliability
Internal consistency estimates were determined from an analysis of test variance using the Kuder-Richardson method. The coefficients ranged from .45 to .95. The test-retest (five-month interval) reliabilities for the subtests range from .28 to .89.

Validity
The test is designed for use within an educational setting and is constructed to have a high face validity within this framework. Test scores correlate poorly with Stanford-Binet scores.

Norms
The norm group of 962 "white, middle-American" children was carefully screened for average intelligence, school achievement in a "middle range," and lack of physical handicaps and emotional disturbances.

Norms for Hearing-Impaired People
None have been established.

Appropriateness for Hearing-Impaired People
Due to the sophisticated English-language component of this test, it would seem inappropriate to use the full-scale ITPA with many hearing-impaired children. The visual sequential memory, visual reception, manual expression, visual closure, and visual association subtests, however, appear appropriate for hearing-impaired children (Weiss, Goodwin, & Moores, 1975).

Range of Scores
For each subtest the raw scores range from 0 to 50. The subtest raw scores represent the sum of the number of creditable responses given on that subtest. Norm tables of psycholinguistic age, psycholinguistic quotient, and scaled equivalents are presented in the manual.

Interpretation
Normative data enables the examiner to derive age equivalents and scaled scores, giving an objective point of reference to judge individual performance in any of the 12 abilities tested.

Summary of Buros Institute Publications

Discussed in the seventh edition of Buros's *Mental Measurements Yearbook* (Vol. 1, pp. 814–825). The ITPA provides a limited measure of conservation. The test emphasizes intra-individual, rather than inter-individual, differences. The standardized group has a "middle-America" bias, with minority groups clearly underrepresented. Much research is still needed before confident statements can be made concerning validity. Nevertheless, the test is carefully constructed and does much to extend the psychometrist's ability to diagnose learning difficulties effectively.

General References

Bateman, B. D. *Interpretation of the 1961 Illinois Test of Psycholinguistic Abilities*. Seattle: Special Child Publications, 1968.

Osgood, C. E. A behaviorist analysis. In J. S. Bruner (Ed.), *Contemporary approaches to cognition*. Cambridge: Harvard University Press, 1957.

References Related to Hearing-Impaired People

Hamlin, C. S. *A study using the Illinois Test of Psycholinguistic Abilities in the determination of the language abilities of hearing-impaired children*. Unpublished master's thesis, University of Kansas, 1963.

Hanson, G. H., Hancock, B. B., & Kopra, L. L. *Relationships among audiological status, linguistic skills, visual-motor perception, and academic achievement of deaf children*. Washington, D.C.: U.S. Department of Health, Education, and Welfare, 1969.

Jaeckel, L. R. *A study in the comparison of teachers' ratings and the Illinois Test of Psycholinguistic Abilities in determining the language ability of deaf and hard of hearing children*. Unpublished master's thesis, University of Kansas, 1963.

Weiss, K., Goodwin, M., & Moores, D. *Evaluation of programs for hearing-impaired children: 1969–1974* (Research, Development and Demonstration Center in Education of Handicapped Children, Research Report No. 91). Minneapolis: University of Minnesota, 1975.

3
INTELLIGENCE TESTS

CATTELL INFANT INTELLIGENCE SCALE

Author
P. Cattell

Publisher
The Psychological Corporation
757 Third Avenue
New York, NY 10017

Price
$160.50 per complete kit (material, carrying case, 25 record forms)

Date of Edition
1960

General Purpose
The purpose of the Cattell Infant Intelligence Scale (CIIS) is to estimate the mental development of infants.

Description
The CIIS is divided into 19 sublevels. These are categorized according to age from two months to 36 months. There are subtopics within each sublevel measuring attention, eye coordination, muscular control, and general responses to objects.

Administration
The CIIS is designed to be administered individually. It should be administered by a person with a sound background in child psychology, including mental testing of school children. The mother may be present during the examination if the infant is shy. There are no time limits for each of the subtests. Few if any verbal instructions are given to the infant (one-word instructions only). Some of the instructions deal with verbal or vocal references. The total time required ranges from 45 to 60 minutes.

Special Administration Procedures for Hearing-Impaired People

No special administration procedures for hearing-impaired children have been established. Caution should be used in administering the CIIS with a hearing-impaired child. The examiner would need to eliminate or account for the voice response babbling and attending to voice subtopics for most hearing-impaired infants.

Age Level

2 to 36 months

Reliability

The reliability of the CIIS was tested using the split-half method corrected by the Spearman-Brown formula. Reliablity scores for the sublevels are high, ranging from .85 to .90, except for reliability coefficients of .56 and .71 for the ages of three months and 36 months, respectively.

Validity

Concurrent validity studies between the different sublevels of the CIIS and Form L of the Stanford-Binet produced correlations ranging from .10 to .87; the lower correlations of .10, .34, .18, and .56 were for three, six, nine, and 12 months, respectively. Validity coefficients for ages 12 months and 36 months ranged from .67 to .83.

Norms

The standardization of the developmental and intelligence scales was obtained at the Center for Research in Child Health and Development, Harvard University. Results of 223 children (113 boys and 110 girls) were used for the final norm tables.

Norms for Hearing-Impaired People

None have been established.

Appropriateness for Hearing-Impaired People

Since a number of the subtopics focus on auditory development and auditory functioning, the test may be inappropriate for many hearing-impaired infants. The validity of an intelligence quotient obtained on a hearing-impaired infant would be questionable using this test. Caution must be exercised in interpreting results.

Range of Scores

The principle of scoring the CIIS is the same as that of the Stanford-Binet Intelligence Test. All items are scored plus or minus. Once a basal score is established, the age score is added with other partial age scores received in higher age categories. The sum of these scores provides a mental age score.

Interpretation

The mental age score of the CIIS can assist a diagnostician in determining the mental development of an infant. The CIIS scores should be used with caution, especially at the earlier levels, due to the low reliability and validity of the test. Misdiagnosis or an undetected diagnosis of handicapping conditions prior to testing can severely affect the results of the test. A complete physical examination should precede the test.

Summary of Buros Institute Publications

Reviewed in the eighth edition of Buros's *Mental Measurements Yearbook* (Vol. 1, pp. 296-297). The reviewers state that the CIIS has provided useful results in several longitudinal research studies and that examiners already committed to its use might profitably continue with it—particularly if they have accumulated a useful set of local norms. However, the reviewers state that some reevaluations of Cattell's standardization and scoring methods might be indicated.

General References

Cattell, P. *The measurement of intelligence of infants and young children.* New York: The Psychological Corporation, 1960.

Society for Research in Child Health and Development. *Center for Research in Child Health and Development of the Harvard School of Public Health* (Publication No. 1). Washington, D.C.: Author, 1960.

Terman, L. M., & Merrill, M. *Measuring intelligence.* Boston: Houghton Mifflin, 1937.

References Related to Hearing-Impaired People

None available

COLUMBIA MENTAL MATURITY SCALE

Author
B. B. Burgemeister, L. H. Blum, and I. Lorge

Publisher
Harcourt Brace Jovanovich, Inc.
757 Third Avenue
New York, NY 10017

Price
$98.00 per kit (cards and manual)
$123.00 per kit plus carrying case
$8.50 per package (35 record forms)

Date of Edition
1972

General Purpose
The purpose of the Columbia Mental Maturity Scale (CMMS) is to measure general reasoning abilities of children. This test helps school personnel select appropriate curriculum materials and learning tasks for children including those who are culturally disadvantaged and physically handicapped.

Description
The CMMS consists of 92 pictorial and figural classification items arranged in a series of eight overlapping scales or levels. Between 51 and 65 items are actually presented, depending upon the level being administered. Children are given levels appropriate for their chronological age. Each item consists of a series of three to five drawings printed on a 6-by-19-inch card. The child is asked to look at all the pictures on the card and to select the one which is different from the others, indicating his/her choice by pointing to it. The items are arranged in approximate order of difficulty.

Administration
The CMMS is administered individually. The test takes 15 to 20 minutes, which includes teaching the child the task, using three sample items, presenting the test items included in the level appropriate for the child's chronological age, and recording his/her response to each item on the Individual Record Form.

Special Administration Procedures for Hearing-Impaired People
No special administration procedures for hearing-impaired people have been established. If necessary, sign language or pantomime may be used to communicate instructions.

Age Level
3 years, 9 months through 9 years, 11 months

Reliability
The median split-half reliability coefficients ranged from .85 to .91 for all test levels. A median test-retest reliability coefficient of .85 was obtained for three different age groups, with an average gain of 4.6 points in the Age Deviation Score (ADS) on the retest. The standard error of measurement is about five ADS points for children 3½ to 5½ years of age and about six ADS points for children 6 to 9½ years of age.

Validity
Results on the CMMS were compared with results from the Stanford-Binet Intelligence Scale (Form L-M) and yielded a correlation coefficient of .67 Results on the CMMS were also compared with results on the Otis-Lennon Mental Ability Test and yielded a correlation coefficient of .69.

Norms
The 1970 national standardization program was designed to yield a stratified quota sample of 2,600 children ages 3 years, 6 months through 9 years, 11 months who were representative of the total population of the United States. The age range was divided into 13 six-month age groups. Two hundred people in each age group were used for developing norms. One-half of the children in each age group were boys and one-half were girls. Each geographic region of the United States was represented. Community size, race, and parental occupations were also taken into account.

Norms for Hearing-Impaired People
None have been established.

Appropriateness for Hearing-Impaired People

As long as the instructions for the test are understood, the test appears to be appropriate for hearing-impaired children. For each item, the child is asked to look at all the pictures and point to the picture that is different from the others on that card. The test items themselves do not discriminate against anyone possessing a hearing problem.

Range of Scores

Raw scores are converted into Age Deviation Scores (ADS). The ADS may be converted to a percentile, stanine, or verbal description. In addition, the total raw score may be converted to a maturity index which can match the child's score with an average score for one of the six-month age groups.

Interpretation

Results may be used for class placement, prescriptive educational programming, and/or remedial service planning.

Summary of Buros Institute Publications

The CMMS is reviewed in the eighth edition of Buros's *Mental Measurements Yearbook* (Vol. 1, pp. 297–302). The reviewers state that the CMMS is a well-constructed and well-normed measure of reasoning ability of young children. It is easy to administer and the manual is complete. It ranks as one of the best assessment techniques for preschool children.

General References

Corwin, B. J. The influence of culture and language on performance of individual ability tests. *Journal of School Psychology*, 1965, *3*, 41–47.

Goldstein, L. S., Coller, A. R., Dill, J., & Tilis, H. S. The effect of a special curriculum for disadvantaged children on test-retest reliabilities of three standardized instruments. *Journal of Educational Measurements*, 1970, *7*, 171–174.

Kanfer, F. H., Durefeldt, P. H., Martin, B., & Dorsey, T. E. Effects of model reinforcement, expectation to perform, and task performance on model observation. *Journal of Personality and Social Psychology*, 1971, *20*, 214–217.

Miller, B. *A comparison of the Columbia Mental Maturity Scale, the Leiter International Performance Scale, and the Wright Short Form of the Stanford-Binet (Form L-M) with the Full Scale Stanford-Binet (Form L-M) on a group of trainable retardates.* Unpublished master's thesis, Central Missouri State College, 1967.

References Related to Hearing-Impaired People

Frey, J. H. *A study of the feasibility of using the Columbia Mental Maturity Scale to predict school achievement of young deaf children.* Unpublished master's thesis, University of Tennessee, 1969.

Kodman, F., Waters, J. E., & Clifford, C. I. Psychometric appraisal of deaf children using the Columbia Mental Maturity Scale. *Journal of Speech and Hearing Disorders*, 1962, *27*, 275–279.

DENVER DEVELOPMENTAL SCREENING TEST

Author
W. K. Frankenburg and J. D. Dodds

Publisher
Ladoca Project and Publishing Foundation, Inc.
East 51st Street and Lincoln Street
Denver, CO 80216

Price
$10.50 (test kit)
$3.25 (100 test forms)
$6.25 (reference manual)
$9.50 (manual workbook)

Date of Edition
1975

General Purpose
The Denver Developmental Screening Test (DDST) is a standardized tool designed as an aid in the early detection of delayed development in children.

Description
The DDST consists of 105 items arranged in four sections. *Personal-Social* tasks indicate the child's ability to get along with people and take care of himself or herself; *Fine Motor-Adaptive* tasks indicate the child's ability to see and use his/her hands to pick up objects and to draw; *Language* tasks indicate the child's ability to hear, carry out commands, and speak; and *Gross Motor* tasks indicate the child's ability to sit, walk, and jump.

Administration
The DDST is designed to be administered individually. The number of items administered varies according to the age of the child. The DDST may be administered with or without the parents. Generally, each section of the test is continued until the child has three failures in each of the four test sections. The total time required is one hour.

Special Administration Procedures for Hearing-Impaired People
No special administration procedures for hearing-impaired people have been established.

Age Level
2 weeks to 6 years

Reliability
Twenty children ranging from 2 months to 5½ years old were tested twice by the same examiner at an interval of one week. The test-retest reliability scores ranged from 90 to 100 percent. The revised scoring test-retest methods yielded 97 percent agreement on test results of 186 children between the ages of 1.5 months and 6.3 years.

Validity
Correlations ranging from .74 to .97 were obtained from 236 children who were evaluated with the DDST and either the Stanford-Binet Intelligence Test or the Bayley Scale for Infants Test.

Norms
The DDST was standardized on 1,036 (543 male, 493 female) "normal" Denver, Colorado, children between the ages of two weeks and 6.4 years. Children who were adopted, premature, or known to be handicapped in any way were excluded from the sample.

Norms for Hearing-Impaired People
None have been established.

Appropriateness for Hearing-Impaired People
For older hearing-impaired children, this test may be administered by use of sign language, pantomime, or demonstration, if necessary. The only section of the DDST that would not be appropriate for hearing-impaired individuals, regardless of age, is the language section.

Range of Scores
When a child fails any item that 90 percent of the children normally can pass at a younger age, this is considered a delay in development. Items are scored in terms of pass, fail, refusal, and no opportunity for the child to perform the item.

Interpretation

The DDST is interpreted in categories of normal, questionable, abnormal, and untestable, based on the number of delays on each test. Delays are used to interpret the total DDST results.

Summary of Buros Institute Publications

The DDST is discussed in the seventh edition of Buros's *Mental Measurements Yearbook* (Vol. 1, pp. 733–736). The reviewers question the reliability, validity, and sensitivity of the DDST. They question the geographical selection of the sample as well as the applicability of the norms. The DDST appears to be most valid as a screening technique for children 4 to 4½ years old.

General References

Frankenburg, W. K., & Dodds, J. B. The Denver Developmental Screening Test. *Journal of Pediatrics*, 1967, *71*, 181.

Frankenburg, W. K., Goldstein, A., & Camp, B. W. The revised Denver Developmental Screening Test: Its accuracy as a screening instrument. *Journal of Pediatrics*, 1971, *79*, 988.

References Related to Hearing-Impaired People

None available

HAPTIC INTELLIGENCE SCALE FOR ADULT BLIND

Author

H. C. Shurrager and P. S. Shurrager

Publisher

Stoelting Company
1350 S. Kostner Avenue
Chicago, IL 60623

Price

$435.00 (set of testing materials)
$17.00 (manual)
$11.00 (package of 100 record forms)

Date of Edition

1964

General Purpose

The Haptic Intelligence Scale for Adult Blind (HIS) is a nonverbal test designed to measure the intelligence of blind or partially sighted adults.

Description

The HIS is made up of six subtests: *digit symbol, object assembly, block design, object completion, pattern board,* and *bead arithmetic.* The digit symbol subtest consists of a plastic plate which has simple, raised-up geometric forms. On each form there are raised dots. The individual must touch these designs with one hand and then with the other hand, simultaneously touch each of the 40 problem forms, and tell how many dots correspond with each form. The object assembly subtest consists of four wooden items which must be assembled: a doll, a block, a hand, and a ball. The block design subtest consists of four 1½-inch cubes. The individual has to arrange these cubes so that the top sides match the patterns on templates made from identical materials. The object completion subtest has items which are missing something. The client must discover what is missing by manipulating the item. The pattern board subtest consists of a 7½-inch board with 25 round holes. These holes are arranged in rows of fives. In the center of the board is a fixed peg. Pegs can be inserted in the holes to form patterns. The individual examines the patterns with his/her fingers, then the pegs are withdrawn and the student must reproduce the pattern from memory. The bead arithmetic subtest involves using an abacus. The individual must read numbers off the abacus. The numbers begin with one digit and increase in difficulty until the student is adding numbers of four digits to numbers of three digits.

Administration

The HIS is administered individually and requires up to two hours to complete.

Special Administration Procedures for Hearing-Impaired People

No special administration procedures for hearing-impaired people have been established. When this test is used with a deaf-blind person, the instructions should be given in a mode of communication appropriate to that person.

Age Level

16 to 64 years

Reliability

A test-retest procedure using 136 people resulted in reliability coefficients from .70 to .81. Test-retest reliability for the sum of five subtests (bead arithmetic omitted) was .91. The total IQs from HIS showed a split-half reliability of .95.

Validity

When utilized with the adult blind (ages 20 to 34), the HIS correlation with the Wechsler Adult Intelligence Scale verbal section was .65.

Norms

The individuals in the standardization sample were between the ages of 16 and 64. They represented four designated geographic regions within the United States: Northeast, North Central, South, and West. Visual acuity did not exceed 5/200 in the better eye with correction. Whites and nonwhites, males and females, were included in the sample. No deaf-blind individuals were included.

Norms for Hearing-Impaired People

No norms for hearing-impaired people are available. However, this test has been used effectively with deaf-blind people.

Appropriateness for Hearing-Impaired People

All subtests appear adaptable for use with deaf-blind people.

Range of Scores

Raw scores are converted to scaled scores with a mean of 10 and a standard deviation of three for each subtest. An intelligence quotient may then be obtained from the sum of scaled scores.

Interpretation

The HIS may be used to assist educators or rehabilitation workers with decisions regarding educational and vocational placement and training.

Summary of Buros Institute Publications

Discussed in the seventh edition of Buros's *Mental Measurements Yearbook* (Vol. 1, pp. 737-738). The reviewers state that the HIS is not a perfected test in its present form and should be administered and interpreted with caution. The subtests are interesting. The administration time is long and should be divided into two sessions.

General References

Eber, H. W. Factor structure of WAIS verbal and HIS test combined. *Journal of Educational Research*, 1967, *61*, 27-28.

Kamin, H. S. Onset and duration of blindness: Affectors of Haptic Intelligence Scale Performance. Unpublished doctoral dissertation, Illinois Institute of Technology, 1964.

Saxon, J. P. Comparison of HIS & WAIS on blind psychotics. *Rehabilitation Counseling Bulletin*, 1969, *13*, 49-51.

References Related to Hearing-Impaired People

Vernon, M., Bair, R., & Lotz, S. Psychological evaluation and testing of children who are deaf-blind. *School Psychology Digest*, 1979, *8*(3), 291-295.

Vernon, M., & Green, D. A guide to the psychological assessment of deaf-blind adults. *Journal of Visual Impairment and Blindness*, June 1980, *74*, 229-231.

Hiskey-Nebraska Test of Learning Aptitude

Author
M. S. Hiskey

Publisher
Marshall S. Hiskey
5640 Baldwin
Lincoln, NB 68507

Price
$68.00 (set of testing materials)
$4.00 (50 record booklets)
$2.00 (50 drawing sheets)

Date of Edition
1966

General Purpose
The Hiskey-Nebraska Test of Learning Aptitude (H-NTLA) is a performance test designed for hearing-impaired youth. It measures learning aptitude. Marshall Hiskey does not equate learning aptitude with intelligence. Yet, when the H-NTLA is used with hearing-impaired people, the results are often reported as indicators of general intelligence.

Description
The H-NTLA consists of 12 subtests: *bead patterns, memory for color, picture identification, picture association, paper folding, visual attention span, block pattern, completion of drawings, memory for digits, puzzle blocks, picture analogies,* and *spatial reasoning.* Instructions for each subtest are in the manual. The test may be given to hearing-impaired and normal-hearing individuals.

Administration
The H-NTLA is designed to be administered individually. Testing should take place in a small, familiar room. Personal information such as name, age, grade, and school should be obtained and filled in at the top of the record blank along with the date of the test and the examiner's name. Tests should be given according to the directions, which are derived from preliminary tryouts and have been used in the standardization process. Specific instructions are provided for each student. The total time required ranges from 30 to 45 minutes.

Special Administration Procedures for Hearing-Impaired People
The H-NTLA was designed for hearing-impaired people. Instructions are specific and utilize demonstration and/or pantomime.

Age Level
3 to 17 years

Reliability
Using the split-half method and the Spearman-Brown formula, the coefficients of reliability for 3–10-year-olds were .947 (deaf children) and .933 (hearing children). For 11–17-year-olds, the reliability coefficients were .918 (deaf children) and .904 (hearing children).

Validity
Correlations between the H-NTLA and the Stanford-Binet Intelligence Test, Wechsler Intelligence Scale for Children, Leiter, and other scales for various samples of deaf, mentally retarded, and bilingual children range from the .70s to the .90s.

Norms
Norms are based only on children already given the Stanford-Binet by competent examiners and already classified in the normal range (90 to 110) on that test. This infrequently used procedure seeks to ensure a test population of relatively average children at different age levels. The test was administered to more than 400 children ages four to ten; the children were from midwestern states, primarily Illinois, Nebraska, and Minnesota.

Norms for Hearing-Impaired People

A revised scale was standardized on hearing-impaired children and youth between 2.6 and 17.5 years old. Final sample norms were based on 1,079 hearing-impaired children in ten widely separated states, from New York to Utah to Florida. The majority of children came from state residential schools for the deaf. Most of the children from these schools who fell within specified age groups were tested. The procedure gave a representative sample of hearing-impaired children at each age level.

Appropriateness for Hearing-Impaired People

The H-NTLA is appropriate for most hearing-impaired people. The H-NTLA is often used with hearing-impaired people as a measure of learning aptitude because (1) the test has special instructions for administering the test to hearing-impaired people; (2) there are norms for hearing-impaired children and adolescents; and (3) all test items are performance tasks.

Range of Scores

Raw scores for hearing children are converted to Deviation Intelligence Quotients. The IQ scores range from 36 to 148 with a mean of 100 and a standard deviation of 16. Hearing-impaired children's raw scores are converted to a "learning age." Learning ages range from 3 to 18½ years.

Interpretation

The major interpretive score for deaf children is the learning age. In addition, a learning quotient can be determined by dividing the learning age by the chronological age. The yearly gain in learning ability for hearing-impaired children begins to decrease after age 12; by age 16 the gain is very slight. Chronological age beyond 16, therefore, is considered a constant when computing the learning quotient. (The Deviation IQ norms for hearing children can be found in Table X, page 50 in the instruction manual; the learning age norms for deaf children are on the back page of the record booklet.)

Summary of Buros Institute Publications

As discussed in the eighth edition of Buros's *Mental Measurements Yearbook* (Vol. 1, pp. 307-308), the H-NTLA is a nonverbal measure of mental ability. The test was found to be helpful in the intellectual assessment of a variety of language-handicapped children and youth. Representative comments in a survey show a variety of opinions: no time pressures; gives learning quotient rather than pure IQ; too time-consuming; children score too high; the test consistently ranked behind the Wechsler scale in over-all use. This division of opinion suggests that the manual be read carefully before deciding about the appropriateness of the Hiskey-Nebraska test.

General References

Hiskey, M. S. Norms for children with hearing for the Hiskey-Nebraska Test of Learning Aptitude. *Journal of Educational Research*, 1957, *2*, 137-142.

References Related to Hearing-Impaired People

Giangreco, J. C. *The Hiskey-Nebraska Test of Learning Aptitude as predictor of academic achievement of deaf children.* Unpublished doctoral dissertation, University of Nebraska, 1965.

Hiskey, M. S. A new performance test for young deaf children. *Education and Psychological Measurement*, 1941, *1*, 77-84.

Hiskey, M. S. Measuring mental competence levels of young deaf children. *Volta Review*, 1950, *52*(8), 349-357 (part 1); and 1950, *52*(9), 406-411 (part 2).

KNOX CUBE TEST
Arthur Revision

Author
G. Arthur

Publisher
Stoelting Company
1350 S. Kostner Avenue
Chicago, IL 60623

Price
$11.00 per test kit

Date of Edition
1947 (revised form of Arthur Performance Point Scale)

General Purpose
The Knox Cube Test (KCT) is a subtest of the Grace Arthur Point Scale of Performance (GAPSP). It is a performance test of visual memory span and visual attention span. The entire GAPSP is designed to furnish an intelligence measure for hearing-impaired children, children with reading disabilities, and non-English speaking children.

Description
The KCT consists of four 1-inch cubes fastened 2 inches apart on a base 10½-inches long, 1½-inches wide, and ¼-inch thick. Two pencils must be provided for the student to reproduce a sequence of taps presented initially by the examiner.

Administration
The KCT should be administered individually. The test has two trials, administered at the beginning and end of a test battery. Without using words, the examiner taps a series of blocks with the pencil in a predetermined sequence, then indicates silently that the child is to reproduce the sequence of taps. Several examples may be given until the child has successfully completed the 18 series of taps, or until he/she has failed three series in succession. The total time required is 20 minutes.

Special Administration Procedures for Hearing-Impaired People
The test was designed for hearing-impaired people; no words are necessary in its administration.

Age Level
4½ to 15½ years (according to Arthur manual)

Reliability
No reliability coefficients for the KCT alone are presented.

Validity
No validity studies on the KCT alone are available.

Norms
The entire scale of GAPSP norms was based on students ages 4½ to 15½ years. As the norm group for comparing the Arthur Scale and Binet Intelligence Test results, the author used 968 testees from "middle-class American schools" and a study of 94 persons of the type frequently seen in psychological settings. Age norms are charted in the manual.

Norms for Hearing-Impaired People
No norms for hearing-impaired people are available. However, Bishop (1936) reports results of a study using the GAPSP for deaf and hard-of-hearing children. Goetzinger and Rousey (1957) report KCT findings of 91 deaf students between the ages of 14 and 21 years from a residential school. The reported mean score was 16.2 (two trials) with a standard deviation of 3.0. The authors state that from these results, no conclusions can be drawn relative to retardation of hearing-impaired people in visual memory span.

Appropriateness for Hearing-Impaired People
Although this performance test was designed for use with a hearing-impaired population, it lacks substantial norms for this group. Such norms should be established before it can be a truly effective assessment tool. Bishop (1936) encouraged continued use of the scale with hearing-impaired children. Bonham (1963) concluded that the KCT is "the single best predictor of success in the development of word-recognition skills and oral language in deaf children in the elementary grades."

Range of Scores

The raw score for the test is the average of the two trials. Raw scores may be converted to mental ages using a chart in the manual. Bishop (1936), in a study of 90 hearing-impaired children, reported IQs on the Arthur Scale ranging from 68 to 158 with a mean of 97.

Interpretation

Bonham (1963) relates KCT scores to success in the development of word recognition skills in deaf children in the elementary grades.

Summary of Buros Institute Publications

The KCT by itself is not reviewed by Buros. The fourth edition of Buros's *Mental Measurements Yearbook* (pp. 435-437) does review the GAPSP. The reviewers state that the GAPSP is a fairly reliable measure of intelligence but needs further validation studies.

General References

Arthur, G. *A Point Scale of Performance Test, Revised Form-II, manual for administering and scoring the test.* New York: The Psychological Corporation, 1947.

Hamilton, M. E. A comparison of the Revised Arthur Performance Tests (Form II) and the 1937 Binet. *Journal of Consulting Psychology*, 1949, *13*, 44-49.

Patterson, R. M. Analysis of practice effect on readministration of the Grace Arthur Scale in relation to academic achievement of mentally deficient children. *American Journal of Mental Deficiency*, 1948, *52*, 337-341.

References Related to Hearing-Impaired People

Bishop, H. Performance scale tests applied to deaf and hard-of-hearing children. *Volta Review*, 1936, *38*, 447; 484-485.

Bonham, S. J. *Predicting achievement for deaf children.* Columbus: Ohio Department of Education, 1963.

Goetzinger, C. P., & Rousey, C. L. A study of the Wechsler Performance Scale (Form II) and the Knox Cube Test with adolescents. *American Annals of the Deaf*, 1957, *102*(5), 388-398.

Guthrie, J. T., & Goldberg, H. K. Visual sequential memory ability. *Journal of Learning Disabilities*, 1972, *5*, 102-103.

Kohs Block Design Test

Author
S. C. Kohs

Publisher
Stoelting Company
1350 S. Kostner Avenue
Chicago, IL 60623

Price
$49.50 per complete kit (test, manual, record forms)

Date of Edition
1919

General Purpose
The Kohs Block Design Test (KBDT) is designed to measure intelligence.

Description
The KBDT consists of 16 one-inch-square cubes, whose sides vary in color or combination of two colors. There are also 17 cards containing a specific design. The designs are graded in difficulty by modifying the designs. The client must reproduce the designs using the blocks.

Administration
The KBDT is designed to be administered individually. The examiner displays a design and the person reproduces the design within specified time limits. The time and the number of moves required to complete the design are recorded by the examiner. Each separate and distinct change in the position of a block is counted as a move. The total time required ranges from 30 to 45 minutes.

Special Administration Procedures for Hearing-Impaired People
No special administration procedures for hearing-impaired people have been established. The manual provides for the administration of the test to people either who do not know the names of colors or who cannot understand spoken language. Procedures can be demonstrated through gestures and pantomime.

Age Level
3 to 19 years

Reliability
No information is presented in the manual.

Validity
The correlation between the Binet mental age and the KBDT mental age is .80. Other correlations are: Binet mental age and block design mental age for "feebleminded" cases, .67; and Binet intelligence quotient and block design intelligence quotient, .80.

Norms
The normative sample consisted of 291 public school students and 75 "feebleminded" persons. The manual does not describe the selection process for the normative group nor provide any data pertaining to sex, socioeconomic level, age, or geographic sampling procedures.

Norms for Hearing-Impaired People
The general normative sample included a cross-section of students from the Saskatchewan School for the Deaf, with all grades represented.

Appropriateness for Hearing-Impaired People
The KBDT manual states that valid results may be obtained independent of the language factor, and that neither deafness nor lack of language understanding should limit test performance.

Range of Scores
Raw scores are converted to scaled scores and mental ages. The KBDT reports scaled scores ranging from 0 to 131; conversion to mental age yields a range from 3 years to 19 years, 11 months.

Interpretation
Kohs's intelligence quotient and/or mental age can be used for purposes of educational and vocational placement or prescriptive educational planning.

Summary of Buros Institute Publications
Discussed in the 1940 edition of Buros's *Mental Measurements Yearbook* (pp. 198-199). The reviewer comments that the KBDT is a satisfactory diagnostic tool with some limitations.

General References

Berry, J. W. Ecological and cultural factors in spatial perceptual development. *Journal of Behavioral Science*, 1971, *3*(4), 324-336.

Kosc, L. Kohs test and its qualitative analysis in psychological clinical practice. *Studia Psychologica* (Czechoslovakia), 1966, *8*(3), 241-244.

Larson, R. K. *The Kohs Block Design Test as a diagnostic tool in the area of remedial reading.* Unpublished master's thesis, Moorehead State College, 1964.

Shrivastava, R. Kohs Block Design Test norms for children. *Indian Philosophical Review*, 1967, *4*, 68-70.

References Related to Hearing-Impaired People

Luzski, W. A., & Luzski, M. B. Habilitation suggestions for deaf retarded persons. *Hearing and Speech News*, 1966, *34*(3), 5-7.

McCrone, W.P. Learned helplessness and level of underachievement among deaf adolescents. *Psychology in the Schools*, 1979, *16*(3), 430-434.

LEITER INTERNATIONAL PERFORMANCE SCALE

Author
R. G. Leiter

Publisher
Western Psychological Services
12031 Wilshire Boulevard
Los Angeles, CA 90025

Price
$545.00 per complete kit (trays 1-3, carrying case, 25 record cards, and manual)

Date of Edition
1948

General Purpose
The Leiter International Performance Scale (LIPS) and its revision, the Arthur Adaptation, were developed to provide a culture-free, nonverbal method of assessing general intelligence.

Description
The LIPS is a performance test requiring a person to match various wooden blocks with pictures, ranging from simple pairing of colors and shapes to analyzing complex analogies. The LIPS consists of a series of short subtests subdivided by intellectual age (an average of four subtests per intellectual age).

Administration
The LIPS is an individually administered test developed originally for children who cannot hear. The examiner is encouraged not to communicate with the child during the administration of the test. The child should not be hurried; except for a few block design subtests, all subtests are untimed. The test is usually administered in 30 to 45 minutes.

Special Administration Procedures for Hearing-Impaired People
The LIPS instructions may be demonstrated. Verbal communication is neither permitted nor necessary.

Age Level

2 to 18 years (The Arthur Adaptation is designed for ages 2 to 8.)

Reliability

Split-half reliabilities ranging from .91 to .94 have been reported in several studies of the LIPS.

Validity

Ten reported correlation studies of the LIPS with the Stanford-Binet Intelligence Test yielded a median correlation of .77. Five reported studies of the LIPS and the Wechsler Performance Scales yielded correlations ranging from .75 to .85.

Norms

Information on the norms for LIPS is minimal. The original norm group consisted of Chinese and Japanese children living in Hawaii. When the LIPS was given to children in the continental United States, however, the data from the original norm group were no longer sufficient. Adjustments were made in calculating intelligence quotient scores for children in the continental United States by adding five points to the overall intelligence quotient score.

Norms for Hearing-Impaired People

None have been established.

Appropriateness for Hearing-Impaired People

The test was originally designed for hearing-impaired children. The greatest use of the LIPS has been with multihandicapped hearing-impaired children who are unable to take other established intelligence tests. The test has also been found successful with bilingual children and children suffering from articulatory disorders and cerebral palsy.

Range of Scores

Raw scores are converted to mental ages and intelligence quotients. The mean IQ for the LIPS is 95 with a standard deviation of 16.

Interpretation

Combining the information derived from the LIPS with that from other instruments can help in the development of individualized educational plans. However, because of the discrepancies found in the validity results, caution should be exercised when using the LIPS as the sole criterion for educational placement.

Summary of Buros Institute Publications

Discussed in the sixth edition of Buros's *Mental Measurements Yearbook* (pp. 814-816). The reviewers recommend that additional research be conducted on comprehensive norms and a better scoring system. In addition, cross-cultural research with young children is encouraged. The reviewers feel the LIPS is a very promising instrument.

General References

Leiter, R. G. *Performance tests for measuring native intelligence.* Unpublished master's thesis, University of Southern California, 1929.

Sharp, H. A note on the reliability of the Leiter International Performance Scale (1948 Revision). *Journal of Consulting Psychology*, 1958, *22*, 320.

References Related to Hearing-Impaired People

Birch, J. R., & Birch, J. W. Predicting school achievement in young deaf children. *American Annals of the Deaf*, 1956, *101*, 348-352.

Clegg, S. J., & White, W. F. Assessment of general intelligence of Negro deaf children in a public residential school for the deaf. *Journal of Clinical Psychology*, 1966, *22*, 93-94.

Varva, F. I. *An investigation of the effect of auditory deficiency upon performance with special reference to concrete and abstract tasks.* Unpublished doctoral dissertation, University of Pittsburgh, 1956.

REVISED BETA EXAMINATION

Author
C. E. Kellogg and N. W. Morton

Publisher
The Psychological Corporation
737 Third Avenue
New York, NY 10017

Price
$10.25 (set of 25 test booklets)
$40.00 (set of 100 test booklets)
$2.50 (specimen set)

Date of Edition
1957

General Purpose
The Revised Beta Examination (RBE) is a revision of the U. S. Army Group Examination Beta developed during World War I. It is designed to measure general intellectual ability of persons who are illiterate or non-English speaking.

Description
The RBE is designed as one booklet containing six subtests: *mazes, digit-symbol substitution, error recognition, paper-form board, picture completion*, and *identities*. Specific examples are presented with each subtest to show the examinee how to work through the section.

Administration
The RBE may be administered individually or to a group. For a group, the room should be large enough to allow a separation of at least two feet between the examinees. The examiner can repeat the instructions and review the examples as many times as necessary. An individual testing situation is necessary when an examinee cannot keep pace with group instructions. The directions for individual administration remain the same. Timing varies for each of the six subtests; the full test requires about 40 minutes.

Special Administration Procedures for Hearing-Impaired People
No special administration procedures for hearing-impaired people have been established. However, the precautions mentioned in the instruction booklet applying to all foreign-speaking populations is relevant; repetition of the instructions is encouraged.

Age Level
16 to 59 years

Reliability
A reliability coefficient of .90 was derived from the intercorrelation among subtests used with a standardization group. Two other coefficients of .81 ($N=199$) and .75 ($N=104$) were obtained by correlating the weighted scores on three odd-numbered subtests with three even-numbered subtests.

Validity
Two correlations are given to establish validity. A coefficient of .92 based upon 168 adults is reported between the RBE and the Wechsler-Bellevue Intelligence Scale; a coefficient of .71 based on 198 adults is reported between the RBE and the Otis Self-Administering Test of Mental Ability.

Norms
Norms are based on the performance of 1,225 white, adult, male prisoners at the U. S. Federal Penitentiary at Lewisburg, Pennsylvania. They ranged in age from 16 to 59. The sample was selected so that education and socioeconomic status represented that of the distribution of white, male adults in the 1940 U.S. Census. No females were included in the standardization of norms.

Norms for Hearing-Impaired People
None have been established.

Appropriateness for Hearing-Impaired People
This test was developed for use with persons who speak languages other than English. Theoretically one can include hearing-impaired people in this category.

Range of Scores

Raw scores are converted to scaled scores ranging from 52 to 135 with a mean of 90.6 and standard deviation of 9.8. An answer key is available for partial scoring.

Interpretation

The examiner takes the examinee's score and age and refers to Table II in the instruction booklet to determine the Beta IQ. The Beta IQ is similar in statistical meaning to the Wechsler IQ. The graduated values of the Beta IQs are classified: defective (70 and below), inferior (71-79), below average (80-89), average (90-109), above average (110-119), superior (120-128), and very superior (129 and above).

Summary of Buros Institute Publications

Discussed in the sixth edition of Buros's *Mental Measurements Yearbook* (pp. 769-771). The reviewers are critical of the RBE's validity and reliability studies, especially the limited norm group. They recommend further research before extensive use is made of the RBE.

General References

Bennett, G. K., & Wesman, A. G. Industrial test norms for a southern plant population. *Journal of Applied Psychology*, 1947, *31*, 241-246.

Kellogg, C. E., & Morton, N. W. Revised Beta Examination. *Personnel Journal*, 1934, *13*, 98-99.

Lindner, R. M., & Gurvitz, M. Restandardization of the Revised Beta Examination to yield the Wechsler type of I. Q. *Journal of Applied Psychology*, 1946, *30*, 649-658.

References Related to Hearing-Impaired People

Bolton, B. An alternative solution for the factor analysis of communication skills and nonverbal abilities of deaf clients. *Education and Psychological Measurement*, 1973, *33*(2), 459-463.

Johnson, O.G. Testing the educational and psychological development of exceptional children. *Review of Educational Research*, 1968, *38*(1), 61-70.

SLOSSON INTELLIGENCE TEST

Author
R. L. Slosson

Publisher
Slosson Educational Publications, Inc.
P. O. Box 280
Buffalo Street
East Aurora, NY 14052

Price
$25.00 per kit

Date of Edition
1981 (revised)

General Purpose

The Slosson Intelligence Test (SIT) is described as a brief individual screening instrument designed to assess intelligence.

Description

The format of the SIT emphasizes easy administration and scoring. Correct responses are given unambiguously and are immediately available during testing. Test items are designed for three age-levels: infants (0.5 to 24 months), preschool (two to four years), and above four years. The last two levels require verbal responses.

Administration

The SIT is designed to be administered individually. Different performance requirements are requested from different age groups. Postural control and locomotion are assessed through observation for infants up to 24 months of age. Questions and commands are presented to children between ages 2 and 4. Individuals 4 years of age and older are presented with verbal questions. Regardless of age, the test should take 10 to 30 minutes to complete.

Special Administration Procedures for Hearing-Impaired People

No special administration procedures for hearing-impaired people have been established.

Age Level
2 weeks to adulthood

Reliability
A test-retest (within a two-month interval) reliability coefficient of .97 was reported for a heterogeneous sample of 139 people between ages 4 and 50. The standard error of measurement for the SIT is 4.3.

Validity
The only validity study reported in the manual shows correlations between the SIT intelligence quotients and Stanford-Binet (Form L-M) Intelligence Test. These correlations range from .90 for age four to .98 for ages six and seven.

Norms
The manual does not provide numbers of people within the norm group nor procedures for selection of the sample. Children within the sample were from nursery, public, parochial, and private schools in and around New York City. The population included retarded as well as gifted children. The adults, also from New York state, were chosen from the general population, professional groups, a graduate school, a county jail, and a state school for mentally retarded people.

Norms for Hearing-Impaired People
None have been established.

Appropriateness for Hearing-Impaired People
While it would be possible to administer the SIT to hearing-impaired infants, its use with hearing-impaired people above two years of age appears to be inappropriate because of the heavy emphasis on language skills.

Range of Scores
Raw scores are converted to mental ages, reported in years and months, and scaled-score IQs ranging from 30 to 200.

Interpretation
The results of the SIT are used to help evaluate an individual's mental ability. The SIT reading test gives a "comfortable" reading grade-level from "primer into high school."

Summary of Buros Institute Publications
Discussed in Buros's *Intelligence Tests and Reviews* (pp. 951–954). The reviewers are critical of the test. They state that the heavy emphasis on language skills makes it a difficult test for children who, for cultural or individual reasons, have language problems. The reviewers believe, however, that the SIT may be useful as a quick screening device. It is noted that more research is needed with larger samples of more typical individuals.

General References
DeLapa, G. The Slosson Intelligence Test: A screening and retesting technique for slow learners. *Journal of School Psychology*, 1968, 6, 224–225. (Abstract)

Fagert, C. *The relationship between the Slosson Intelligence Test and the Wechsler Intelligence Scale for Children.* Unpublished master's thesis, Kent State University, 1968.

Kaufman, H., & Ivanoff, J. The Slosson Intelligence Test as a screening instrument with a rehabilitation population. *Exceptional Children*, 1969, 35(9), 745.

References Related to Hearing-Impaired People
None available

Raven's Progressive Matrices

Author
J. C. Raven

Publisher
The Psychological Corporation
757 Third Avenue
New York, NY 10017

Price
$6.10 Progressive Standard Matrices, per copy (Sets A, B, C, D, & E)
$5.00 Coloured Progressive Matrices, per copy (Sets A, AB, & B)
$3.75 Progressive Advanced Matrices, per copy (Set I)
$8.50 Progressive Advanced Matrices, per copy (Set II)

Date of Edition
Progressive Standard Matrices (Sets A, B, C, D, & E): 1938 (revised 1956)
Coloured Progressive Matrices (Sets A, AB, & B): 1947 (revised 1965)
Advanced Progressive Matrices (Set I: 1943; Set II: 1962)

General Purpose
The Raven's Progressive Matrices (RPM) was developed in England to provide a measure of intelligence through an individual's capacity for observation and clear thinking.

Description
Each form of the RPM consists of 60 matrices or designs. The individual chooses a missing insert of a matrix from six or eight alternatives. The items are grouped into five series, each containing 12 matrices of increasing difficulty. Different forms are suggested for specific age groups and educational levels.

Administration
The RPM may be administered individually or to a group. Everyone, regardless of age, is given the same series of problems in the same order and is asked to work at his/her own speed, without interruption. Very simple oral instructions are required. There is no time limit. The test may be completed in about 30 minutes.

Special Administration Procedures for Hearing-Impaired People
No special administration procedures for hearing-impaired people have been established. Instructions can be effectively communicated in sign language, gestures, or demonstrations and can be repeated until thoroughly comprehended.

Age Level
8 to 65 years (Progressive Standard Matrices)
5 to 11 years (Coloured Progressive Matrices)
Adolescents and adults (Advanced Progressive Matrices)

Reliability
Reliability coefficients of .83 to .93 were derived using a test-retest method on groups of older children and adults who were moderately homogeneous in ages. Reliability coefficients for scores tend to be lower for the very young and very old.

Validity
Criterion-based validity with both verbal and performance parts of the tests range between .40 to .75, tending to be higher with performance than with verbal tests. Studies with mentally retarded and different occupational and educational groups indicate fair concurrent validity. Predictive validity coefficients using academic criteria run somewhat lower than those of the usual verbal intelligence tests.

Norms
Norms are provided for each half-year interval between eight and 14 years of age, and for each five-year interval between 20 and 65 years of age. The norms are based on British samples, including 1,407 children; 3,665 men in military service tested during World War II; and 2,192 civilian adults.

Norms for Hearing-Impaired People

None have been established.

Appropriateness for Hearing-Impaired People

The Coloured Progressive Matrices is designed specifically for individuals who for whatever reason cannot understand or speak the English language. All forms of the RPM have been used successfully with hearing-impaired people.

Range of Scores

The RPM scores are compiled by noting the number of items correctly solved (raw score). This is converted into a percentile based on age-related norms.

Interpretation

A person's total score provides an index of intellectual capacity, whatever the person's nationality or education.

Summary of Buros Institute Publications

Discussed in the fourth edition of Buros's *Mental Measurements Yearbook* (pp. 416-422). Commenting on the standard matrices (Sets A, B, C, D, & E), the reviewers are critical of the validity due to too many poor items and a low general factor between the five sets. They also state that the test is almost a pure "g" test, which usually measures a psychological "thing" rather than predict successful behavior in special social situations. The reviewers suggest that the geometrical matrices are not entirely culture-free and might show discrepancies between those individuals whose jobs require abstract, relational thinking and those whose jobs do not.

In assessing the coloured matrices (Sets A, AB, & B), the reviewers are critical of the undependable reliability of the test for use with very young children. The RPM (Sets I & II) is reported to be a valuable instrument, simply constructed and easily administered.

General References

Foulds, B. A., & Raven, J. C. An experimental survey with progressive matrices. *British Journal of Psychology*, 1950, *20*, 104-110.

References Related to Hearing-Impaired People

Abrol, B. M., Vagrecha, Y. S., & Saxena, K. Assessment of intelligence in the patient population having impairment of hearing. *Indian Journal of Mental Retardation*, 1973, *6*(2), 75-80.

Bolton, B. An alternative solution for the factor analysis of communication skills and nonverbal abilities of deaf clients. *Education and Psychological Measurement*, 1973, *33*(2), 459-463.

Goetzinger, M. R., & Houchins, R. R. Colored Raven's Progressive Matrices with deaf and hearing subjects. *American Annals of the Deaf*, 1969, *114*(2), 95-101.

Hess, D. W. Evaluation of the young deaf adult. *Journal of Rehabilitation of the Deaf*, 1969, *3*(2), 6-21.

STANFORD-BINET INTELLIGENCE SCALE

Author
L. M. Terman and M. A. Merrill

Publisher
Houghton Mifflin Company
1919 S. Highland
Lombard, IL 60148

Price
$99.00 (test materials and manual)

Date of Edition
1973 (third revision of Form L-M with 1972 norms)

General Purpose
The Stanford-Binet Intelligence Scale (S-BIS) is designed to measure a person's present level of "general intelligence."

Description
The basic materials of the S-BIS include: a test manual, a record book for recording responses, two booklets of printed cards, and a box of standard toy objects. The scale itself consists of a single Form L-M. This form is broken down into age levels from two through Superior Adult III. Each level consists of six subtests (with exception of the average adult level, which has eight subtests). Within each level, the subtests are of uniform difficulty and contain items that progressively become harder. One alternate subtest is also provided at each age level. They are used for substitute purposes if the regular subtests are found inappropriate because of special circumstances which interfere with their standardized administration.

Administration
The S-BIS is designed to be administered individually. The examiner should begin testing at a level slightly below the expected mental age of the examinee. The examiner first tests for a level where the individual passes all subtests; this level is called the basal age. Then testing continues upward until a level is obtained where all subtests are failed; this is the ceiling age. Credit is given for all subtest items passed above a basal age and a mental age is determined for the individual. Also provided is an abbreviated scale which consists of four valid and representative subtests in each age level. These should be used when time limits the administration of the entire scale. The total time required ranges from 30 to 90 minutes.

Special Administration Procedures for Hearing-Impaired People
No special administration procedures for hearing-impaired people have been established.

Age Level
2 years and above

Reliability
In general, the reliability coefficients for most of the various age and IQ levels are over .90; these coefficients are derived from measures of internal consistency. This test also "tends to be more reliable for the older than for the younger ages, and for the lower than for the higher IQs" (Anastasi, 1982, p. 237).

Validity
Criterion-related validity, as shown by correlations between the S-BIS and school grades, teacher's ratings, and achievement test scores, mostly falls between .40 and .75. Construct validity is shown by item retention and selection based upon several factors: correlation with mental age on the preceding 1916, 1937, and 1960 forms; age differentiation; and internal consistency indicated by a mean item-scale correlation of .66 for the 1960 revision.

Norms

The 1972 restandardization of Form L-M was based on a more representative sample than the 1937 S-BIS norm group. The new norms were obtained from a sample of approximately 2,100 students tested during the 1971-72 school year. To achieve national representation, the test publishers used students who were part of the large-scale norming for the Cognitive Abilities Test, the Iowa Test of Basic Skills, and the Tests of Academic Progress given in the fall of 1970. These students were included in a selected sample reflecting economic status, race, and ethnic background of residents in representative communities chosen on the basis of population and geographic region.

Norms for Hearing-Impaired People

None have been established.

Appropriateness for Hearing-Impaired People

The S-BIS appears to be an inappropriate and invalid measure of intelligence for most hearing-impaired people. Anastasi (1982, p. 241) points out that the test is "largely a measure of scholastic aptitude" and that it is "heavily loaded with verbal functions, especially at the upper levels. Individuals with a language handicap, as well as those whose strongest abilities lie along nonverbal lines, will thus score relatively low on such a test."

Range of Scores

Raw scores are converted to mental ages and intelligence quotients. The IQ scores range from 30 to 171 with a mean of 100 and a standard deviation of 16.

Interpretation

IQ Score	Classification
140-169	Very superior
120-139	Superior
110-119	High average
90-109	Normal or average
80-89	Low average
70-79	Borderline defective
30-69	Mentally defective

Summary of Buros Institute Publications

Reviewed in the seventh edition of Buros's *Mental Measurements Yearbook* (Vol. 1, pp. 767-773). The reviewer states that his remarks are similar to comments made 32 years ago: "the Stanford-Binet Intelligence Scale is an old, old vehicle. It has led a distinguished life as a pioneer in the bootstrap operation that is the assessment enterprise. Its time is just about over...."

General References

Anastasi, A. *Psychological testing* (5th ed.). New York: Macmillan, 1982.

Concannon, S. J. Comparison of the Stanford-Binet Scale with the Peabody Picture Vocabulary Test. *Journal of Educational Research*, 1975, *69*(3), 104-105.

Terman, L. M., & Merrill, M. A. *Stanford-Binet Intelligence Scale: Manual for the Third Revision, Form L-M* [With revised IQ tables by S. R. Pinneau and 1972 tables of norms by R. L. Thorndike]. Boston: Houghton Mifflin, 1973.

References Related to Hearing-Impaired People

Adler, S. *The non-verbal child*. Springfield, Ill.: Charles C. Thomas Publisher, 1964.

Berlinsky, S. Measurement of the intelligence and personality of the deaf: A review of the literature. *Journal of Speech and Hearing Disorders*, 1952, *17*, 39-54.

Farrant, R. H. The intellective abilities of deaf and hearing children compared by factor analyses. *American Annals of the Deaf*, 1964, *109*(3), 306-325.

Howard, J. O. *A comparison of the revised Stanford-Binet Intelligence Scale, Form L-M, and the Nebraska Test of Learning Aptitude, 1966 revision* [With groups of mentally retarded, deaf, and normal children]. (Unpublished doctoral dissertation, University of New Mexico, 1969). *Dissertation Abstracts International*, 1969, *30*, 3322A.

Osler, S. P. The nature of intelligence. *Volta Review*, 1965, *67*(4), 285-291.

Vernon, M., & Brown, D. W. A guide to psychological tests and testing procedures in the evaluation of deaf and hard-of-hearing children. *Journal of Speech and Hearing Disorders*, 1964, *29*(4), 414-423.

Vineland Social Maturity Scale

Author
E. A. Doll

Publisher
American Guidance Service, Inc.
Publishers Building
Circle Pines, MN 55014

Price
$5.00 (25 test forms)
$3.70 (manual)

Date of Edition
1965

General Purpose
The major purposes of the Vineland Social Maturity Scale (VSMS) are (1) to sample various aspects of social ability such as self-sufficiency, occupational activities, communication, self-direction, and social participation; and (2) to reflect progressive freedom from need of assistance, direction, or supervision by others.

Description
The VSMS is a detailed test showing the progressive capacity of children to look after themselves and to participate in activities which lead toward ultimate independence as adults. The 117 items on the scale are arranged in order of increasing difficulty, representing progressive maturation.

Administration
The VSMS is designed to be administered individually. The items of the VSMS are scored on the basis of information obtained from someone intimately familiar with the person being evaluated, such as the mother, father, or guardian. The examiner completes one item at a time, but notes incidental information relative to other items. In obtaining information, the examiner is expected to quiz the informant in a sympathetic manner, encouraging spontaneous description and eliciting detailed facts. The person being evaluated need not be present or observed. There is no way to ascertain the length of time needed to complete the scale.

Special Administration Procedures for Hearing-Impaired People
No special administration procedures for hearing-impaired people have been established. However, several examiners have used the VSMS with hearing-impaired people by obtaining information through a relative or guardian.

Age Level
Birth to 35 years

Reliability
Systematic data for the evaluation of test-retest reliability are reported on results for "feeble-minded" individuals. Reliability by the split-half method yields a measure only of the consistency of item scaling. There is evidence which indicates high reliability for a single examiner employing different informants for the same individuals without appreciable time intervals between examinations. Additional presumption of reliability may be inferred from the relatively high discriminative values of item and total scores.

Validity
Validity of the scale was reported on "feeble-minded" individuals only. Estimation of a "normal" person's social maturity was reported in terms of the social competence of persons of the same age and sex as the individual.

Norms
Norms are based on performance of ten male and ten female white people for each year of age from birth through 30 years. This results in a norm group of 620 persons divided equally by sex and age. All these people lived in the Greater Vineland area of Cumberland County in southern New Jersey. Selection of people was influenced by evidence of family economic status, attained school grade, parental school grades, and (if working) occupational classification.

Norms for Hearing-Impaired People
None have been established.

Appropriateness for Hearing-Impaired People
This test may be administered successfully to hearing-impaired people without modification. However, there may be discrepancies in results among examiners due to differences in examining procedures. Also it should be noted that some observational items relate directly to auditory functioning; this should be accounted for in presentation of results. The VSMS has been used successfully in cases where individual testing of a multihandicapped hearing-impaired person with other instruments was impossible.

Range of Scores
Items are grouped into eight categories of adaptive behavior and receive one of the following scores: satisfactorily and habitually performed, item not performed during test due to lack of opportunity, task not performed due to lack of environmental opportunity, task in transitional state, or task not successfully performed. A total score is obtained by adding the basal score (highest of all continuous pluses) and the scattered credits beyond the basal score. The total score is then converted to an age score by interpolation according to year-score values on the record sheet.

The derived age scores may be converted to ratios or quotients. The same procedure is used for converting the Binet mental age scores to intelligence quotients. The social age is statistically and methodologically comparable to Binet's mental age, and the social quotient is comparable to Binet's intelligence quotient.

Interpretation
A final score is to be interpreted with due regard for special limiting circumstances such as physical disability, ill health, sensory defects (including deafness), adult domination, and other barriers. Limitations imposed by factors such as intelligence level, emotional attitudes, social conditioning, and disposition are presumed to be reflected in the scale itself. In general, exceptional circumstances should be recorded under "remarks" and taken into consideration in the interpretation of scores; the scores themselves, however, should be as factually objective as possible. Results may be used to assist educators or social service personnel in educational placement or psycho-social planning.

Summary of Buros Institute Publications
Discussed in the first edition of Buros's *Personality Tests and Reviews* (pp. 470-472, 574-576). The reviewers are critical of the utilization of potentially biased observations by untrained and possibly emotionally involved reporters. The reviewers also suspect the possibility of hearsay reporting rather than direct observation reporting. Nevertheless, the VSMS is a valuable tool if used wisely.

General References
Doll, E. A. The inheritance of social competence. *Journal of Heredity*, 1937, *28*, 153-165.

Doll, E. A. IQ and mental deficiency. *Journal of Consulting Psychology*, 1940, *4*, 53-61.

Pendrini, D. T., & Pendrini, L. N. The Vineland Social Maturity Scale: Recommendations for administration, scoring and analysis. *Journal of School Psychology*, 1966, *5*, 14-20.

References Related to Hearing-Impaired People
Avery, G. Social competence of pre-school acoustically handicapped children. *Exceptional Children*, 1948, *15*, 71-73.

Bradway, K. P. Social competence of exceptional children: The deaf, the blind, and the crippled. *Exceptional Children*, 1937, *4*, 64-69.

Burchard, E. M. L., & Myklebust, H. R. A comparison of congenital and adventitious deafness with respect to its effect on intelligence, personality, and social maturity: Part II, social maturity. *American Annals of the Deaf*, 1942, *87*(2), 140-154.

WECHSLER ADULT INTELLIGENCE SCALE—REVISED

Author
D. Wechsler

Publisher
The Psychological Corporation
757 Third Avenue
New York, NY 10017

Price
$70.00 per set of testing materials (equipment, manual, package of 25 record forms, carrying case)

Date of Edition
1981

General Purpose
The Wechsler Adult Intelligence Scale—Revised (WAIS-R) is an updated edition of the Wechsler Adult Intelligence Scale (WAIS) which was published in 1955. The purpose of the WAIS-R is to measure the intelligence of adults.

Description
The WAIS-R consists of 11 subtests divided into verbal and performance sections. The six subtests in the verbal section are *information*, *comprehension*, *arithmetic*, *similarities*, *digit span*, and *vocabulary*. The five subtests in the performance section are *digit symbol*, *picture completion*, *block design*, *picture arrangement*, and *object assembly*.

Administration
The WAIS-R is designed to be administered individually. The subtests are administered in the order prescribed in the manual. The examiner should always read the instructions and questions from the manual and not try to interpret what is said. Time for the entire test varies from 45 to 60 minutes.

Special Administration Procedures for Hearing-Impaired People
No special administration procedures for hearing-impaired people have been established.

Age Level
16 years, 0 months through 74 years, 11 months

Reliability
For every subtest except digit span and digit symbol, reliability was determined by computing a correlation between scores on odd and even items and by correcting the coefficient for the full test by the Spearman-Brown formula. In addition, the WAIS-R manual reports the following reliability coefficients: .97 for the full scale, .93 for performance IQ, and .97 for verbal IQ. The standard error of measurement is 2.53 for the full scale, 4.14 for the performance scale, and 2.74 for the verbal scale.

Validity
Validity of the WAIS-R is based on existing data reported in the 1955 edition of the WAIS. One coefficient of .85 based upon 52 adults is reported between the WAIS and the Stanford-Binet Intelligence Test. A coefficient of .72 is reported between the WAIS and the Raven's Progressive Matrices. The author of the WAIS-R believes that validity studies of this new edition will be forthcoming as it replaces the 1955 edition of the WAIS.

Norms
Norms are based on the performance of a stratified sample of 1,880 people selected according to the 1970 U. S. Census and tested between 1976 and 1980. The sample was divided into nine sections by age: 16-17, 18-19, 20-24, 25-34, 35-44, 45-54, 55-64, 65-69, 70-74. The sample was selected according to distribution by age, sex, race (white, nonwhite), geographic region, urban-rural residence, race, occupation, and education.

Norms for Hearing-Impaired People
None have been established.

Appropriateness for Hearing-Impaired People

The WAIS-R verbal scale is an inappropriate intelligence measure for many hearing-impaired adults. People who cannot fully comprehend spoken words would be unable to take a number of the verbal subtests. Sign language would be inappropriate because of lack of standardization in vocabulary. The performance scale, however, is an excellent test for use with most hearing-impaired clients. Instructions can be demonstrated or presented using sign language. The WAIS-R is ideally used along with a supplementary performance intelligence measure. In using the performance section as a sole measure of intelligence, one cannot infer that the quantitative result measures verbal intelligence.

Range of Scores

Raw scores are converted to intelligence quotients and scaled scores. The WAIS-R full-scaled intelligence scores range from 45 to 150 with a mean of 100 and a standard deviation of 15. For each of the 11 subtests the scaled scores range from 1 through 19 with a mean of 10 and a standard deviation of three. A table is provided which equates full-scaled scores with intelligence quotients.

Interpretation

The IQ scores are clustered into seven descriptive labels of intellectual ability as follows:

IQ Score	Classification
130 & above	very superior
120-129	superior
110-119	bright normal
90-109	average
80-89	dull normal
70-79	borderline
69 & below	mental defective

Summary of Buros Institute Publications

The WAIS-R has not yet been reviewed in Buros's *Mental Measurements Yearbooks*. The WAIS was reviewed in the seventh edition of the yearbook (Vol. 1, pp. 776-790). The reviewers indicate that the WAIS is the best adult, individual intelligence test available.

General References

Boor, M. Relationship of test anxiety and academic performance when controlled for intelligence. *Journal of Clinical Psychology*, 1972, *28*(2), 171-172.

Dickstein, L. S., & Kephart, J. L. Effect of explicit examiner expectancy upon WAIS performance. *Psychological Reports*, 1972, *30*(1), 207-212.

Matarazzo, J. *Wechsler's measurement and appraisal of adult intelligence*. New York: Macmillan, 1972.

Matarazzo, R. G., Weins, A. N., Matarazzo, J. D., & Manaugh, T. S. Test-retest reliability of the WAIS in a normal population. *Journal of Clinical Psychology*, 1973, *29*(2), 194-197.

References Related to Hearing-Impaired People

Brill, R. G. The superior IQ's of deaf children of deaf parents. *Journal of Rehabilitation of the Deaf*, 1970, *4*(20), 45-53.

Goetzinger, C. P., & Rousey, C. L. A study of the Wechsler Performance Scale (Form 2) and the Knox Cube Test with deaf adolescents. *American Annals of the Deaf*, 1957, *102*(5), 388-398.

Lehman, J. U., & Simmons, M. P. Comparison of rubella and non-rubella young deaf adults: Implications for learning. *Journal of Speech and Hearing Research*, 1972, *15*(4), 734-742.

WECHSLER INTELLIGENCE SCALE FOR CHILDREN—REVISED

Author
D. Wechsler

Publisher
The Psychological Corporation
757 Third Avenue
New York, NY 10017

Price
$80.50 per set of testing materials (equipment, manual, 25 record forms, carrying case)
$10.50 per manual
$23.00 per package of 100 record forms

Date of Edition
1974

General Purpose
The Wechsler Intelligence Scale for Children—Revised (WISC-R) battery is a revision of the original Wechsler Intelligence Scale for Children, which was developed to provide a reliable measure of intellectual functioning. The WISC-R has established itself as a useful clinical and diagnostic tool in the areas of educational assessment and appraisal of learning and other disabilities.

Description
The WISC-R is made up of five verbal subtests (*information, similarities, arithmetic, vocabulary,* and *comprehension*) and five performance subtests (*picture completion, picture arrangement, block design, object assembly,* and *coding*). There also are one optional verbal subtest (digit span) and one optional performance subtest (mazes) that may be substituted for one or two of the regular subtests.

Administration
The WISC-R is designed to be administered individually. Instructions are presented verbally for all subtests. For the verbal section, the examiner is requested not to change the phrasing of test items, spell words, or provide additional assistance. The administration of the WISC-R requires a friendly relationship between examiner and child, properly organized materials, and sufficient time to give the test in an easy manner. The verbal and performance tests are alternated to make the testing session more interesting and varied. The total time required to administer the full battery ranges from 50 to 75 minutes.

Special Administration Procedures for Hearing-Impaired People
No procedures for administration of the WISC-R to hearing-impaired children are presented by the author. Special administration procedures for the performance subtests of the WISC-R, developed by Ray (1979), are outlined in the next review.

Age Level
6 to 16 years

Reliability
The verbal, performance, and full-scale IQs have high reliabilities across all age ranges; the average coefficients are .94, .90, and .96, respectively. The reliabilities for the individual subtests are quite satisfactory, with average coefficients ranging from .77 to .86 for the verbal subtests and from .70 to .85 for the performance subtests.

Validity
Three correlations are provided to establish validity. A coefficient of .82 was found between the WISC-R full-scale IQ and the Wechsler Preschool and Primary Scale of Intelligence (WPPSI) full-scale IQ. A coefficient of .95 was found between the WISC-R and WAIS full scales. The correlation between the WISC-R and WAIS verbal IQs is .96 and the correlation between the WISC-R and WAIS performance IQs is .83. Correlation coefficients of .71, .60, and .73 were found between the Stanford-Binet Intelligence Test and the WISC-R verbal, performance, and full scale, respectively.

Norms
Norms for the WISC-R were derived using a stratified sampling plan to ensure that the normative sample of 2,200 people would include representative proportions of various classes of children in the United States. The stratification along selected variables was arranged in accordance with the 1970 U. S. Census. The variables were age,

sex, race (white, nonwhite), geographic region, occupation of head of household, and urban-rural residence.

Norms for Hearing-Impaired People

In a study conducted by Anderson and Sisco (1977), the performance scale of the WISC-R was standardized on a national sample of 1,228 deaf children. Data were collected from 18 residential schools and 4 day-schools for deaf children located throughout the United States. The characteristics of the deaf sample were similar to those of the WISC-R hearing sample. Information concerning the hearing status of the parents and the communication method used during testing is reported. The mean WISC-R performance IQ for the deaf sample is 95 with a standard deviation of 18. Norms for hearing-impaired children have also been gathered by Ray (1979) and will be discussed in the next review.

Appropriateness for Hearing-Impaired People

The WISC-R verbal scale appears to be an inappropriate intelligence measure for most hearing-impaired children. The performance scale, however, is an excellent test for use with many school-age, hearing-impaired children. Only the performance intelligence quotient is reported for most hearing-impaired individuals. Caution should be exercised in using this limited result as an indicator of over-all intellectual ability.

Range of Scores

Raw scores are converted to intelligence quotients and scaled scores. The WISC-R full-scale IQ ranges from scale scores of 41 through 179 with a mean of 100 and a standard deviation of 15. For each of the 12 subtests, scaled scores range from 1 to 19 with a mean of 10 and a standard deviation of 3.

Interpretation

IQ Scores (Full, Verbal, Performance)	Category
130 & above	very superior
120–129	superior
110–119	high average
90–109	average
80–89	low average
70–79	borderline
69 & below	mentally deficient

Summary of Buros Institute Publications

Discussed in the eighth edition of Buros's *Mental Measurements Yearbook* (Vol. 1, pp. 337–355). According to the reviewers, the standardization procedure of the WISC-R has been altered sufficiently to include a proportional representation of nonwhite children in the normative sample. Reliability coefficients are as high or higher than for the WISC, and the coefficients are now given for all age groups rather than only three as in the original version. The WISC-R manual gives no criterion-related, predictive validity data despite the intensive validity research available.

General References

Anastasi, A. *Psychological testing* (5th ed.). New York: Collier Macmillan, 1982.

Glasser, A. J., & Zimmerman, I. L. *Clinical interpretation of the Wechsler Intelligence Scale for Children (WISC)*. New York: Grune & Stratton, 1967.

Sattler, J. M. *Assessment of children's intelligence*. Philadelphia: W. B. Sanders Co., 1974.

References Related to Hearing-Impaired People

Anderson, R., & Sisco, R. Standardization of the WISC-R Performance Scale for deaf children (Office of Demographic Studies publication, Series T, No. 1). Washington, D.C.: Gallaudet College, 1977.

Brill, R. G. The relationship of Wechsler IQs to academic achievement among deaf students. *Exceptional Children*, 1962, *28*(6), 315–321.

Evans, L. A comparative study of the Wechsler Intelligence Scale for Children (Performance) and Raven's Progressive Matrices with deaf children. *The Teacher of the Deaf*, 1966, *64*, 76–82.

Hirshoren, A., Hurley, O., & Hunt, J. The WISC-R and the Hiskey-Nebraska test with deaf children. *American Annals of the Deaf*, 1977, *122*(4), 392–394.

Ray, S. *An Adaptation of the Weschler Intelligence Scale for Children—Revised for the Deaf*. Natchitoches, La.: Northwestern State University of Louisiana, 1979.

An Adaptation of the Wechsler Intelligence Scale for Children—Revised for the Deaf

Author
S. Ray

Publisher
Dr. Steven Ray
Northwestern State University of Louisiana
P. O. Box 5003
Natchitoches, LA 71457

Price
$30.00 per kit (does not include the WISC-R test itself)

Date of Edition
1979

General Purpose
The WISC-R Adaptation was developed to aid psychologists in providing an adequate assessment of a hearing-impaired child's intelligence using the WISC-R Performance Scales.

Description
The WISC-R Adaptation contains a manual (with supplemental and alternate instructions) and supplemental items for each of the WISC-R performance subtests. The instructions closely follow those prescribed by Wechsler except that the linguistic level has been lowered to make the instructions more comprehensible to the general population of deaf children ages 6 to 16. This was deemed necessary for standardization of procedures.

Administration
Not relevant

Special Administration Procedures for Hearing-Impaired People
As described by Ray (1979), the WISC-R in the past was administered through total communication to 91.7 percent of the deaf testees, through an oral method (speech only) to 7.4 percent of the testees, and through fingerspelling with speech to .8 percent of the testees. In the WISC-R Adaptation, standardized instructions are provided for all performance subtests regardless of mode of communication used.

Age Level
6 to 16 years

Reliability
The author assumes that the reliability of his adaptation is the same as the WISC-R because no test items were changed.

Validity
Summary statistics of 127 protocols of hearing-impaired children are presented in the manual. A T-test was performed on the overall performance IQ (PIQ) to determine if the scores obtained differed significantly from those expected for hearing children. The mean PIQ resulting from the adaptation was 99.25 with a standard deviation of 19.35; this compares with the Wechsler norms which have a mean of 100 and a standard deviation of 15. The T-value resulting from a comparison of these scores indicates that the mean PIQs of hearing-impaired children probably do not differ from the mean PIQs of hearing children.

Norms
Not relevant

Norms for Hearing-Impaired People
One hundred and twenty-five hearing-impaired people were used in the norming sample for the WISC-R Adaptation. In general, the author attempted to approximate closely those components of the original WISC-R sample relative to distribution by sex, race, geographic region, and parental occupation.

Appropriateness for Hearing-Impaired People

The WISC-R Adaptation is designed specifically for use with hearing-impaired children. The attempt to standardize procedures and include practice items for performance subtests improves the validity of results obtained on hearing-impaired children. The total time required ranges from 30 to 45 minutes.

Range of Scores

The mean and standard deviation (SD) for each performance intelligence subtest as well as the mean and SD for the PIQ are as follows:

Subtest	Mean	SD
Picture Completion	9.90	3.22
Picture Arrangement	9.28	3.85
Block Design	9.81	3.48
Object Assembly	10.71	3.43
Coding	9.32	3.46
PIQ	99.25	19.35

Interpretation

The WISC-R Adaptation is more accurate than WISC-R itself, because it provides bases for comparing a hearing-impaired child's intellectual functioning not only with other hearing-impaired children but also with hearing children.

Summary of Buros Institute Publications

Not presently reviewed in Buros's *Mental Measurements Yearbooks*

General References

Not applicable

References Related to Hearing-Impaired People

Ray, S. *An Adaptation of the Wechsler Intelligence Scale for Children—Revised for the Deaf.* Natchitoches, La.: Northwestern State University of Louisiana, 1979.

4
PERSONALITY TESTS

BALTHAZAR SCALES OF ADAPTIVE BEHAVIOR I & II

Author
E. E. Balthazar

Publisher
Consulting Psychologists Press, Inc.
577 College Avenue
Palo Alto, CA 94306

Price
Specimen I: $5.00
Specimen II: $8.75

Date of Edition
1973

General Purpose

The Balthazar Scales of Adaptive Behavior (BSAB) is designed to provide a system for program development and evaluation and social behavior assessment among profoundly and severely mentally-retarded adults and mildly retarded youngsters.

Description

There are two major sections of the BSAB scales. The BSAB I focuses on functional independence, including eight ratings: eating, dependent feeding, finger foods, spoon usage, fork usage, drinking, total dressing, and toileting. The BSAB II focuses on social adaption, including 19 ratings grouped in seven categories: unadaptive self-directed behavior (five ratings), adaptive self-directed behaviors (one rating), adaptive interpersonal behavior (three ratings), communication (two ratings), play activities (three ratings), response to instructions (three ratings), and personal care and other behaviors (two ratings).

Administration

The BSAB is designed to be administered individually and in the testee's natural environment. The individual is observed while engaged in typical daily activities. Checklists and numerical scales are provided for rating behaviors. The scale involves frequency counts per unit in time. There is no way to estimate the total time required to complete the scales.

Special Administration Procedures for Hearing-Impaired People

No special administration procedures for hearing-impaired people have been established. Rating methods include observation of the individual in his/her natural environment or interviews with staff members who are familiar with the person.

Age Level

Profoundly and severely retarded adults and mildly retarded youngsters

Reliability

Inter-rater reliability scores are provided for each of the scales. The reliability coefficients range from .43 to .95.

Validity

Validity statistics are not provided in the manual.

Norms

Persons using the BSAB are encouraged to undertake independent studies to obtain descriptive data regarding particular populations or groups of individuals. The only population study listed in the manual provides the mean scores of ambulant people who are profoundly or severely retarded.

Norms for Hearing-Impaired People

None have been established.

Appropriateness for Hearing-Impaired People

The BSAB I functional independence rating scales are appropriate for scoring behaviors of severely or profoundly mentally retarded hearing-impaired individuals. The BSAB II scales of adaptive behavior would require some modification, and the rater would need to understand the individual's mode of communication. This is especially true for the social vocalizations subtest.

Range of Scores

Raw scores are recorded by tallying all the subscale behaviors on the appropriate sections of the tally sheet during each rating session. Raw scores are then transcribed to the scoring summary sheet.

Interpretation

The manual suggests graphing or diagramming, especially when the profile scores are to be studied by groups for program design, inservice training, and research.

Summary of Buros Institute Publications

Reviewed in the eighth edition of Buros's *Mental Measurements Yearbook* (Vol. 1, pp. 695-699). The reviewers state that the BSAB scales are thorough survey instruments which can provide a wealth of information. This information can contribute significantly to the delivery of programs and services to the individual. Other definite pluses are the handbooks and the manual. One weakness is the author's assumption that the usual ward or cottage person can handle the intricate and highly subjective rating schemes. As a whole, the BSAB may be one of the best tools for improving the adaptive and social functioning of the profoundly and severely retarded.

General References

Balthazar, E. E., & English, G. E. A factorial study of unstructured ward behaviors. *American Journal of Mental Deficiencies*, 1969, *3*, 353-360.

Balthazar, E. E., & English, G. E. A system for the social classification of the more severely mentally retarded. *American Journal of Mental Deficiencies*, 1969, *3*, 363-368.

References Related to Hearing-Impaired People

None available

CALIFORNIA PSYCHOLOGICAL INVENTORY

Author
H. G. Gough

Publisher
Consulting Psychologists Press, Inc.
577 College Avenue
Palo Alto, CA 94306

Price
$8.50 (25 booklets)
$3.25 (manual)
$12.50 (scoring key)

Date of Edition
1975 (revised)

General Purpose
The California Psychological Inventory (CPI) is designed for assessing characteristics of personality which have wide applicability to normal human behavior. The CPI measures specific variables concerning the following 18 standard scales: dominance, capacity for status, sociability, social presence, self-acceptance, sense of well-being, responsibility, socialization, self-control, tolerance, good impression, communality, achievement via conformance, achievement via independence, intellectual efficiency, psychological-mindedness, flexibility, and femininity.

Description
The CPI consists of 408 items that relate to the 18 scales in the test. The individual taking the test answers true or false to descriptive statements applied to himself/herself. Items may not be answered at the individual's discretion.

Administration
The CPI may be administered individually or to a group. The test is primarily self-administered; however, individuals are asked to read directions aloud. The examiner may define vocabulary in question, but each testee should use his/her own judgment for concepts not clearly understood. Reliability indicates that the CPI can be administered in formal, informal, and take-home settings with little variance in scoring. Total time required ranges from 45 to 60 minutes.

Special Administration Procedures for Hearing-Impaired People
No guidelines are provided to indicate special administration procedures for hearing-impaired people. The vocabulary of test items may inhibit some prelingually deaf individuals from understanding the context of the questions.

Age Level
High school through adulthood (12 to 65 years)

Reliability
Reliability coefficients are given for each of the 18 scales in the test. They range from .38 to .87, with two scales falling below .59 (communality and psychological mindedness).

Validity
Validity coefficients in the test manual use criteria ratings of staff and educators applied to college and high school students. Coefficients range from .21 to .57 among the 18 scales. No concurrent validity is available.

Norms
The data were developed from consolidation of available samples into a single composite score for each sex. Standard scores were thus derived from samples of 6,200 males and 7,150 females. Sample selection was determined by age, socioeconomic status, and geographic area.

Norms for Hearing-Impaired People
None have been established.

Appropriateness for Hearing-Impaired People
Because the CPI is verbally based, it appears to be inappropriate for use with most hearing-impaired people.

Range of Scores
Raw scores are converted to standard scores. The standard scores for the 18 scales are plotted on a linear graph ranging from 0 to 100 with a mean of 50.

Interpretation

General profile score range, unique profile features, and the internal variability of an individual's profile are means of interpretating scores to clients.

Summary of Buros Institute Publications

Discussed in the eighth edition of Buros's *Mental Measurements Yearbook* (Vol. 1, pp. 518-522). Research has shown that the CPI can help select talented youth and predict delinquent behavior. Areas of further research include the development of behavioral profiles and types, exploration of correlates of scale interactions, influence of demographic variables, and updated validity sources. Clients have no difficulty understanding the meaning of high, average, or low scores on the various scales.

General References

Gault, U. Three short factor scales from the California Psychological Inventory. *Journal of Counseling and Clinical Psychology*, 1975, *43*(5), 274.

Mitchell, J., & Pierce-Jones, J. A factor analysis of Gough's California Psychological Inventory. *Journal of Counseling Psychology*, 1960, *24*(5), 453-456.

Stroup, A., & Manders-Cheid, R. The California Psychological Inventory: Reappraisal of reliability. *Journal of General Psychology*, 1975, *92*, 217-224.

References Related to Hearing-Impaired People

None specifically relevant; however, of related interest:

Pollock, J. *Linguistic performance and personality in high school students*. Unpublished doctoral dissertation, New York University, 1972.

Schwartzentruber, A. *Personality predictors of communication skills*. Unpublished doctoral dissertation, University of British Columbia, 1976.

CALIFORNIA TEST OF PERSONALITY

Author

E. W. Tiegs, W. W. Clark, and L. P. Thorpe

Publisher

California Test Bureau
Del Monte Research Park
Monterey, CA 93940

Price

$12.95 (package of 35 tests)
$8.50 (package of 50 answer sheets)
$3.85 (IBM scoring stencil)

Date of Edition

1953

General Purpose

The California Test of Personality (CTP) is designed to measure the personal and social adjustment patterns of individuals.

Description

The CTP is designed as a booklet and requires yes or no answers to 180 questions. There are two alternate forms, Form AA and BB. Answers to questions are grouped into two major subtests, personal adjustment and social adjustment.

Administration

The CTP may be administered individually or to a group. Pencils must be supplied. Examinees can record responses in the test booklet or on separate answer sheets. Individuals are requested to answer all questions. There are no strict time limits. Three sets of directions are given: "for pupils who are too immature either to read the questions or to mark their answers in the test booklet;" "for 2nd and 3rd graders who need it read to them but can mark their own answers;" and "for more mature pupils who can both read the questions and mark the answers." The total time required ranges from 45 to 60 minutes.

Special Administration Procedures for Hearing-Impaired People

No special administration procedures for hearing-impaired people have been established. However, the directions as presented in the manual for a poor reader may be applied to a hearing-impaired person if it is possible to communicate with that client effectively. If the hearing-impaired person possesses sufficient reading ability (approximately fifth-grade level), he/she should be able to complete the test unaided.

Age Level

Kindergarten to adult

Reliability

Coefficients were computed with the Kuder-Richardson formula. They are given for primary, elementary, intermediate, secondary, and adult levels. This involves an intercorrelation between the personal adjustment and social adjustment subtests. The correlations range from .51 to .83 (primary), .59 to .93 (elementary), .70 to .97 (intermediate), .70 to .91 (secondary), and .66 to .93 (adult) for Forms AA or BB. The correlation coefficients for total adjustment, using both forms, are given as .94, .97, .98, and .97 for the primary, elementary, intermediate, secondary, and adult levels, respectively; the standard error of measurement ranges from 5.38 at the primary level to 9.34 at the adult level.

Validity

The only information provided about validity is written statements from schools using and/or evaluating the test.

Norms for Hearing-Impaired People

None have been established.

Appropriateness for Hearing-Impaired People

Because the CTP depends on language and reading ability, it does not appear to be an appropriate personality measure for a majority of hearing-impaired people. A hearing-impaired person reading at about the fifth-grade level should be able to take this test. Even if an evaluator can communicate via sign language with a client, misunderstanding of the content of the questions may occur.

Range of Scores

Raw scores are converted to percentiles for personal and social adjustment as well as total adjustment.

Interpretation

Norms are listed in the manual to allow for comparison of scores. The results may be used in diagnosis of adjustment problems in school or at work. The results of this test should not be used as a sole criterion for psycho-social program planning.

Summary of Buros Institute Publications

Discussed in the first edition of Buros's *Personality Tests and Reviews* (pp. 721-724). The reviewers state that the 1953 revision of the CTP was probably the result of criticisms by earlier reviewers. Serious doubts are expressed about the revision's usefulness in the selection of employees. However, the review concludes that "in spite of criticism, as personality inventories go, the California test would appear to be among the better ones available."

General References

Lindermann, S. *The effect on scores of individual vs. group administration of the California Test of Personality*. Unpublished master's thesis, Pennsylvania State University, 1954.

Peak, B. *The California Test of Personality: A study of validation*. Unpublished doctoral dissertation, Florida State University, 1963.

Smith, L. The concurrent validity of six personality and adjustment tests for children. *Psychological Monographs*, 1958, 72(4), 1-30.

References Related to Hearing-Impaired People

Horlick, R., and Miller, M. A. A comparative personality study of a group of stutterers and hard-of-hearing patients. *Journal of General Psychology*, 1966, 63, 259-266.

Vegely, A. B., & Elliot, L. L. Applicability of a standardized personality test to a hearing-impaired population. *American Annals of the Deaf*, 1968, 113(4), 858-868.

Devereux Adolescent Behavior Rating Scale

Author
P.E. Haimes, G. Spivack, and J. Spotts

Publisher
The Devereux Foundation Press
Hahnemann Mental Health Center
Hotel Philadelphia
314 N. Broad Street
Philadelphia, PA 19107

Price
$4.50 (25 scales and manual)

Date of Edition
1967

General Purpose
The Devereux Adolescent Behavior Rating Scale (DABRS) is designed to describe the overt behaviors and symptoms which help define a total clinical picture of a disturbed adolescent.

Description
The DABRS is an observational rating scale focusing on 12 behavioral factors: unethical behavior, defiant resistive, domineer sadistic, heterosexual interest, hyperactivity expansive, poor emotional control, needs approval, dependency, emotional distance, physical inferiority timidity, schizoid withdrawal, bizarre speech and cognition, and bizarre action. The scale also includes three behavior clusters such as inability to delay, paranoid thinking, and anxious self blame.

Administration
The DABRS is designed to be administered individually. The scale should be completed by an individual who has intimate knowledge of the adolescent. Rating is done through observation of an adolescent for a two-week period. The instructions for rating are spelled out in detail in the rating manual. Total time required ranges from 10 to 15 minutes.

Special Administration Procedures for Hearing-Impaired People
No special administration procedures for hearing-impaired people have been established. The DABRS may be completed by a person familiar with the adolescent. That person should be knowledgeable about typical hearing-impaired adolescent behavior.

Age Level
13 to 18 years

Reliability
Reliability of the test was established in terms of test-retest and rater-agreement. Using the test-retest method, the median correlation was .82. In rater-reliability, the median correlation was .46 and the mean coefficient of agreement was .90.

Validity
No information provided in the manual

Norms
Norms were derived from research studies which included ratings of 834 institutionalized adolescents, 92 "normal" adolescents in group-living foster homes, and 305 "normal" teenagers living at home with their parents.

Norms for Hearing-Impaired People
None have been established.

Appropriateness for Hearing-Impaired People
Caution must be taken when using the DABRS with a hearing-impaired person. Although the test items do not discriminate against individuals with auditory impairments, interpretation of results can be made only by an evaluator who has knowledge of and experience with hearing-impaired adolescent behavior.

Range of Scores
Raw scores range from 4 to 40.

Interpretation

For each behavioral dimension the manual provides a range of normal scores as well as cut-off scores which indicate clear pathologies. The range of normal scores and cut-off scores differ for each of the behavioral dimensions. Scores can assist parents, counselors, teachers, or psychologists in preparing a treatment program or residential and educational placement.

Summary of Buros Institute Publications

Discussed in the seventh edition of Buros's *Mental Measurements Yearbook* (Vol. 1, pp. 134–135). The reviewers feel that the DABRS is a useful tool in clinical situations as well as research studies. The scale is not useful for making fine discriminations among normal adolescents. However, the instrument can assist in identifying disturbed adolescents.

General References

Spivack, G., Haimes, P. E., & Spotts, J. Adolescent symptomatology and its measurement (Grant No. 1870-P). In *Report to Vocational Rehabilitation Administration*. Washington, D.C.: U.S. Department of Health, Education, and Welfare, 1967.

References Related to Hearing-Impaired People

None available

DRAW-A-PERSON PROJECTIVE TECHNIQUE
Urban's Scoring System

Author
W. H. Urban

Publisher
Western Psychological Services
12031 Wilshire Boulevard
Los Angeles, CA 90025

Price
$22.00 per examiner's kit (25 tests)
$6.50 (25 record booklets)
$6.50 (25 interpretive booklets)
$6.00 (manual)

Date of Edition
1963

General Purpose
Draw-a-Person (DAP) is a projective technique based on the belief that a person will structure a situation corresponding to unique personality dynamics, thereby disclosing important information about himself/herself through the task of drawing a person.

Description
The DAP is a semistructured technique in which the person is instructed to draw male and female figures.

Administration
The DAP is designed to be administered individually. The person is provided a stack of 8½ by 11 white paper and a No. 2, black-lead pencil. The examiner says, "Please draw a picture of a person." The situation is left as unstructured as possible. The examiner observes the behavior of the person and records the uninhibited responses. The person taking the test is to be assured that the test is not of artistic ability. The examiner then asks the person to draw a figure of the opposite sex. Total time required varies greatly.

Special Administration Procedures for Hearing-Impaired People

No special administration procedures for hearing-impaired people have been established. The performance nature of the test lends itself to use with hearing-impaired people.

Age Level

5 years and above

Reliability

No data available

Validity

Statistics not provided in the manual

Norms

None provided

Norms for Hearing-Impaired People

None have been established.

Appropriateness for Hearing-Impaired People

Results are obtained independent of any language factor. The DAP instructions may be administered through sign language, pantomime, or demonstration without upsetting standard administration procedures. The DAP is one of the most frequently used measures of personality with hearing-impaired children, adolescents, and adults.

Range of Scores

Urban's DAP scoring system consists of a four-page interpretative report describing the person's behavior while drawing, a checklist to evaluate possible behaviors and their significance, the examiner's impression of the DAP figures on a 24-graphic-ratings scale, and a comparison of the male and female figures on 10 qualitative dimensions. There are two checklists, the first for severe mental-emotional disturbance and the second for organic brain damage. There are a number of other scoring systems that have been used with the DAP. Most evaluators use no quantitative scoring system, however, relying more on semiprojective, descriptive interpretation of self-concept and interpersonal styles of behavior.

Interpretation

The examiner is to identify areas of conflict, exaggeration, omission, and distortion. The examiner should refer to the descriptive catalog to interpret the major areas of the DAP drawings: head, hands, arms, shoulders, chest, torso, legs, and feet. The final report should also include a description of the person's attitude toward the DAP and differential treatment of male and female figures.

Summary of Buros Institute Publications

According to the seventh edition of Buros's *Mental Measurements Yearbook* (Vol. 1, pp. 401–405), evaluation of the DAP drawing must be done with a variety of other tests and techniques. The DAP should not be used as a primary diagnostic tool of personality. Urban's checklists, providing arbitrary cut-off scores for severity of diagnosis, are presented with no supportive data.

General References

Cauthen, N. R., Sandman, C. A., Kilpatrick, D. G., & Deabler, H. L. DAP correlates of scores on the MMPI. *Journal of Projective Technique and Personality Assessment*, 1969, 9, 262–264.

Ludwig, D. J. Self-perception and the Draw-a-Person test. *Journal of Projective Technique and Personality Assessment*, 1969, 9, 257–261.

Machover, K. *Personality projection in the drawing of the human figure* (8th ed.). Springfield, Ill.: Charles C. Thomas Publisher, 1971.

References Related to Hearing-Impaired People

Bolton, B., Donoghue, R., Langbauer, W. Quantification of two projective tests for deaf clients: A large sample validation study. *Journal of Clinical Psychology*, 1973, 2, 249–250.

Di Leo, J. H. *Children's drawings as diagnostic aids*. New York: Brunner/Mazel, 1973.

HANDICAP PROBLEMS INVENTORY

Author
G. N. Wright and H. H. Remmers

Publisher
Purdue Research Foundation
Purdue University
Lafayette, IN 47907

Price
$4.00 per package (25 tests)

Date of Edition
1960

General Purpose
The Handicap Problems Inventory (HPI) is designed as a measure of self-perceived problems caused by disability.

Description
The HPI is a questionnaire and contains 280 items categorized in four areas: *personal*, *family*, *social*, and *vocational*. The scores represent a quantification of the psychological impact of the disability upon the client as he/she perceives it.

Administration
The test is a structured interview which may be administered individually or to a group. Approximate time required is 30 minutes.

Special Administration Procedures for Hearing-Impaired People
No special administration procedures for hearing-impaired people have been established. Because of the interview format, communication between examiner and client is vital.

Age Level
16 years and above

Reliability
The coefficients of reliability, based on Kuder-Richardson Formula 20, range from .91 to .95 for the four areas.

Validity
No information provided. The manual states that the HPI reflects self-perceptions and indicates that the validity is equivalent to the reliability.

Norms
The norm sample consisted of 1,027 randomly selected, physically disabled clients of the Indiana Division of Vocational Rehabilitation.

Norms for Hearing-Impaired People
None have been established.

Appropriateness for Hearing-Impaired People
The HPI may be an appropriate test for hearing-impaired people if the examiner can conduct a lucid interview in the communication mode of the interviewee. Interpretation of the results should not be made without a thorough understanding of the psycho-social aspects of hearing impairment on personality development.

Range of Scores
Raw scores are converted to percentiles.

Interpretation
Low percentile scores are interpreted in two ways: The client has a tendency to minimize his/her handicap, or the client covers up serious problems.

Summary of Buros Institute Publications
According to the sixth edition of Buros's *Mental Measurements Yearbook* (pp. 237–239), the HPI may be used to assist a counselor in understanding the problems of a disabled client. No test-retest coefficients are reported. The intercorrelation among the four areas is not reported. The reviewer felt that research would be needed to validate the test.

General References

Blaskovics, T. L. *Measurement of the impact of disability upon handicapped persons.* Unpublished doctoral dissertation, University of Wisconsin, 1965.

Hauck, W. E. *The derivation of item weights and additional normative data for the Handicap Problems Inventory.* Unpublished doctoral dissertation, University of Wisconsin, 1968.

Holman, R. J. *Change in self-evaluation of vocational problems among physically, mentally, culturally handicapped clients during the vocational rehabilitation process.* Unpublished doctoral dissertation, University of Wisconsin, 1968.

Koechel, J. W. *Perceptual defense and perceptual vigilance in individuals with obvious and hidden disabilities.* Unpublished doctoral dissertation, University of Houston, 1964.

Lasky, R. G., & Salomone, P. R. A modification of the Handicap Problems Inventory. *Rehabilitation Counseling*, 1971, *15*(2), 106-115.

Matthews, J. B. *The psychological impact of physical disability upon vocationally handicapped individuals.* Unpublished doctoral dissertation, University of Wisconsin, 1966.

Rosillo, R. H., & Fogel, M. L. Emotional support. *Psychosomatic*, 1970, *11*(3), 194-196.

Wright, G. N. *Wisconsin studies in vocational rehabilitation* (2 vols.). Madison: University of Wisconsin (Regional Rehabilitation Research Institute), 1968. (Monograph)

References Related to Hearing-Impaired People

None available

HOUSE-TREE-PERSON PROJECTIVE TECHNIQUE
Buck Scoring System

Author
J. N. Buck

Publisher
Clinical Psychology Publishing Co.
4 Conant Square
Brandon, VT 05733

Price
$4.50 per manual

Date of Edition
1948

General Purpose
The House-Tree-Person Projective Technique (H-T-P) is designed to obtain information concerning the sensitivity, maturity, flexibility, efficiency, and degree of integration of a person's personality. Secondarily, the H-T-P can be used as a measure of intellectual ability.

Description
The client is asked to draw three separate pictures: a house, a tree, and a person. The individual is timed for each task, and the examiner makes notes of the person's behavior or comments during this first phase. In the second phase the client is given an opportunity to define and interpret what was drawn, and the examiner can ask questions.

Administration
The H-T-P may be administered individually or to a group; individual testing is more useful. The client is asked to draw the "best" house, tree, and person, and to take whatever time is necessary. The individual may erase as often as he/she wishes, without penalty, but must complete the drawings freehand, without any other materials. The examiner records the time needed to complete each task and notes the individual's general behavior, comments, sequences of detail, and general tempo. When the drawings are completed, the examiner invites the individual to discuss each drawing. Total time required varies greatly.

Special Administration Procedures for Hearing-Impaired People

No special administration procedures for hearing-impaired people have been established. Minimal knowledge of language is necessary for individuals to complete the first phase of the test. An evaluator's knowledge of sign language would be helpful for some hearing-impaired individuals during discussion of the completed drawings.

Age Level

5 years and above

Reliability

Cannot be judged because of the projective nature of the test

Validity

Cannot be judged because of the projective nature of the test

Norms

Tentative norms for adult intelligence (at least 15 years of age) are provided. One hundred and forty adults representing seven intelligence levels (imbecile, moron, borderline, dull average, average, above average, and superior) were chosen. Adults of the imbecile through average level were white residents of Virginia who were patients or employees of the Lynchburg State Colony. Adults of the above-average group were students of the Universities of Nebraska and Virginia; adults of the superior group were graduate students of the University of Virginia.

Norms for Hearing-Impaired People

None have been established. However, Davis and Hoopes (1976) compared H-T-P drawings of 80 deaf children and 80 hearing children ages 7 to 10. This technique was used to distinguish between children rated by their teachers as poorly adjusted and those rated as well adjusted. No differences were found between hearing-impaired and hearing individuals.

Appropriateness for Hearing-Impaired People

The initial phase of the test is nonverbal and, therefore, appropriate for hearing-impaired people. The second phase of the test should not be attempted if the evaluator cannot carry on a productive and detailed conversation with the person being tested. This may mean a thorough knowledge of sign language on the part of the examiner. The H-T-P is frequently used as a measure of personality with hearing-impaired children, adolescents, and adults.

Range of Scores

A quantitative scoring system was developed by Buck to differentiate between relatively gross classification levels of intelligence. A qualitative system of scoring the drawings was also established by Buck to differentiate between personality adjustment and maladjustment. This system focuses on details, proportion, perspective, time, and comments (spontaneous and induced). As with the Draw-a-Person technique, many evaluators do not use a quantitative scoring system for interpreting results; they prefer a descriptive interpretation of results.

Interpretation

Interpretations of intelligence and personality are based on the degree of distortion or omission in the drawings and on the comments made during and after the test. The scoring system is explained in detail in the manual.

Summary of Buros Institute Publications

Discussed in the fifth edition of Buros's *Mental Measurements Yearbook* (pp. 236-239). The reviewers state that the H-T-P technique is one of the most thorough projective techniques of its type and cannot be properly mastered from manuals and journal articles. Because of flaws in the scoring system, examiners must be cautious about qualitative interpretations.

General References

Buck, J. N. *H-T-P technique: A qualitative and quantitative scoring manual.* Los Angeles: Clinical Psychology Publishing Co., 1948.

Davis, E.E., & Ekwall, E. E. Mode of perception and frustration in reading. *Journal of Learning Disabilities*, 1976, *9*(7), 448–454.

Devore, J. F., & Fryrear, J. L. Analysis of juvenile delinquents hole drawing responses on the tree figure of the House-Tree-Person technique. *Journal of Clinical Psychology*, 1976, *32*(3), 731–736.

Eyal, C., & Lindgren, H. C. The House-Tree-Person test as a measure of intelligence and creativity. *Perceptual and Motor Skills*, 1977, *44*(2), 359–362.

Stavrianos, B. K. Can projective test measures aid in the detection and differential diagnosis of reading deficit? *Journal of Personality Assessment*, 1971, *35*(1), 80–91.

References Related to Hearing-Impaired People

Davis, C. J., & Hoopes, J. L. Comparison of House-Tree-Person drawings of young deaf and hearing children. *School Psychology Digest*, 1976, *5*(2), 29–35.

Donoghue, R. J. Personality development in deaf children as measured by the House-Tree-Person and Bender-Gestalt tests. *Dissertation Abstracts International*, 1975, *35*(10), 5106B.

MEADOW/KENDALL SOCIAL-EMOTIONAL ASSESSMENT INVENTORY

Author
K. P. Meadow

Publisher
Outreach
Pre-College Programs
Gallaudet College
Box 114
Washington, DC 20002

Price
$12.50 (manual and ten forms)
$1.50 (package of ten forms)

Date of Edition
1980

General Purpose
The Meadow/Kendall Social-Emotional Assessment Inventory (SEAI) is designed to identify positive classroom and school behaviors as well as "problem" or "pathological" behaviors of hearing-impaired children and adolescents.

Description
The SEAI consists of 59 questions which are divided into three separate scales: *Social Adjustment* (Scale 1), *Self Image* (Scale 2), and *Emotional Adjustment* (Scale 3).

Administration
The SEAI is designed as an observational rating scale to be completed by a person familiar with the student. The rater should have at least eight weeks of observations with a student prior to completing the inventory. A second rating by a colleague who is familiar with the student may be used to supplement the major evaluator's ratings. The total time required ranges from 20 to 30 minutes.

Special Administration Procedures for Hearing-Impaired People
The SEAI was designed for use with hearing-impaired students.

Age Level

7 to 21 years

Validity

Face validity was confirmed though factor analyses and inspection of items appropriate to hearing-impaired students.

Reliability

The inter-item reliabilities of the three scales are .96 for Scale 1, .94 for Scale 2, and .91 for Scale 3.

Norms

Not relevant

Norms for Hearing-Impaired People

Norms for the SEAI are based on hearing-impaired children from both residential schools and day programs in the northeast, north central, southwest, and southern United States. Three factors were accounted for in the norm distribution: sex, type of educational program, and age group. Using these criteria, 2,071 students were available for establishing norms for Scale 1; 1,757 students for Scale 2; and 2,042 students for Scale 3.

Appropriateness for Hearing-Impaired People

The SEAI is an appropriate behavioral rating scale for hearing-impaired students. The test items were designed specifically with an understanding of the implications of a hearing impairment on normal developmental behavior.

Range of Scores

Raw scores are converted to percentiles based on normative data broken down by age and sex.

Interpretation

Percentiles may be converted into three different ranges: below average, average, and above average. The SEAI should be used as a tool in identifying a student's social and emotional strengths and weaknesses as one develops a plan for an appropriate educational program.

Summary of Buros Institute Publications

The SEAI has not been reviewed in Buros's *Mental Measurements Yearbooks.*

General References

Not relevant

References Related to Hearing-Impaired People

Meadow, K. P. Personality and social development of deaf persons. In B. Bolton (Ed.), *Psychology of deafness for rehabilitation counselors.* Baltimore: University Park Press, 1976.

Mindel, E. D., & Vernon, M. *They grow in silence: The deaf child and his family.* Silver Spring, Md.: National Association of the Deaf, 1971.

Schlesinger, H. S., & Meadow, K. P. *Sound and sign: Childhood deafness and mental health.* Berkeley: University of California Press, 1972.

68 / Assessment of Hearing-Impaired People

MINNESOTA MULTIPHASIC PERSONALITY INVENTORY

Author
S. R. Hathaway and J. C. McKinley

Publisher
The Psychological Corporation
757 Third Avenue
New York, NY 10017

Price
Form R: $6.00 (test booklet); $3.50 (manual)

Group Form: $13.50 (package of 25 tests); $3.50 (manual)

Date of Edition
1967

General Purpose
The Minnesota Multiphasic Personality Inventory (MMPI) is a standardized inventory designed to elicit a wide range of self-descriptions and to provide, in quantitative form, a set of evaluations of an individual's personality status and emotional adjustment.

Description
Each person is asked to answer 566 true or false items as they apply to him/her. The individual's choices are scored on ten scales which purport to give quantitative measures of hypochondriasis, depression, hysteria, psychopathy, paranoia, psychasthenia, masculinity-femininity, schizophrenia, and hypomania.

Administration
The MMPI may be administered individually (Form R) or to a group (Group Form). The examiner should first be sure that the individual comprehends the subject matter. If there is no pre-test evidence, then the first few items can be used to gauge the person's competence. After explaining the general procedures, the examiner can ask the individual to read aloud a few of the items and discuss the reasoning behind the replies. Because of the way the MMPI is scored, any item not marked true or false is, in effect, eliminated from the test. Therefore, every effort should be made to keep the number of unanswered questions to a minimum. Typically, 90 minutes is required to complete either form of the test.

Special Administration Procedures for Hearing-Impaired People
No special administration procedures for hearing-impaired people have been established. The same precautions mentioned for the general administration of the test should be followed for hearing-impaired people.

Age Level
16 years and above, with at least 6 years of successful schooling

Reliability
Reported test-retest reliabilities for six of the ten clinical scales range from .57 to .83.

Validity
Validity measures are reported for single scales between patients of a given diagnosis, unselected patients, and "normals." Satisfactory differentiation is reported in most cases. Many controls which are not present in most personality inventory validation groups, such as cultural factors, patient status, and socioeconomic level are reported for the MMPI.

Norms
The authors gathered a sample of 700 individuals, including "normal" men and women and selected adult patients in clinics of the University of Minnesota Hospitals. The "normal" individuals were friends and relatives of patients who were willing to complete the inventory while sitting in the waiting rooms. They were asked a few background questions to determine their compatibility to the clinical cases in terms of age, education, marital status, occupation, and area of residence. The sample of adults corresponded well in age, sex, and marital status with the 1930 Census of the Minnesota population.

Norms for Hearing-Impaired People

None have been established.

Appropriateness for Hearing-Impaired People

The MMPI is generally inappropriate for use with many hearing-impaired people because it is verbally based and requires good reading skills. If background information about the person and observations of the examiner confirm that the hearing-impaired person comprehends the test's language, the test may be useful.

Range of Scores

Raw scores are converted to T-scores for each of the ten scales with a mean of 50 and a standard deviation of 10. A score above 70 is considered to indicate abnormality.

Interpretation

Interpretations of the MMPI depend heavily upon the individual skill and experience of the psychologist. Substantial knowledge about general personality concepts—in addition to basic understanding of the MMPI and its research literature—is needed before meaningful and useful interpretations can be drawn.

Summary of Buros Institute Publications

Discussed in the eighth edition of Buros's *Mental Measurements Yearbook* (Vol. 1, pp. 907–962). The MMPI is the most extensively researched instrument in personality assessment. Its versatility and power as a predictive instrument is unmatched. The MMPI is *the* objective instrument for the assessment of psychopathology.

General References

Anthony, N. C. Comparison of clients' standard, exaggerated, and matching MMPI profiles. *Journal of Consulting and Clinical Psychology*, 1971, *36*, 100–103.

Dahlstrom, W. G. *Basic readings on the MMPI in psychology and medicine*. Minneapolis: University of Minnesota Press, 1956.

Dahlstrom, W. G., Welsh, G. S., & Dahlstrom, L.E. *An MMPI handbook*. Minneapolis: University of Minnesota Press, 1967.

References Related to Hearing-Impaired People

Rosen, A. Limitations of personality inventories for assessment of deaf children and adults as illustrated by research with the Minnesota Multiphasic Personality Inventory. *Journal of Rehabilitation of the Deaf*, 1967, *1*(2), 47–52.

Rosen, A. *MMPI responses of deaf college preparatory students*. Unpublished monograph, Gallaudet College, 1963.

Tomko, M. A. An analysis of personality profiles obtained on the Minnesota Multiphasic Personality Inventory by deaf and hard-of-hearing adolescents throughout the United States. *Dissertation Abstracts International*, 1974, *34*, (10), 6396A.

RORSCHACH METHOD

Author
H. Rorschach

Publisher
Grune & Stratton, Inc.
111 Fifth Avenue
New York, NY 10003

Price
$32.00 per 10 Rorschach plates

Date of Edition
1921

General Purpose
The Rorschach Method is a projective technique designed to provide an inventory of behavior patterns through stimulation of a person's imagination. The assumption underlining the method is that personality can be assessed on the basis of responses elicited from abstract drawings.

Description
The technique consists of ten nonspecific forms or inkblots which can be shown to the individual on cards or slides.

Administration
The Rorschach may be administered individually or to a group. Individual testing is preferred because of the psychodynamics involved in projective methods. The individual is shown the inkblots one at a time. The examiner asks the client what each form brings to mind. The examiner records the responses of the client, being extremely careful not to influence the individual's responses in any way. After all of the inkblots have been shown, the "inquiry" phase of the technique begins. The examiner asks the individual to point out what part of the blot is being used (area) and what makes him/her see it that way (determinant). The total time required ranges from 45 to 60 minutes.

Special Administration Procedures for Hearing-Impaired People
No special administration procedures for hearing-impaired people have been established. An examiner wishing to use the Rorschach Method with a hearing-impaired individual must be able to communicate effectively with that person; accurate interpretation of a person's response is vital. In most cases, this would mean an examiner who is fluent in American Sign Language. The use of an interpreter would not be recommended because an interpreter's personality might affect the results.

Age Level
3 years and above

Reliability
Reliability of scoring depends to a large extent on the similarity of training of the examiners and has been reported in correlation ranges of .64 to .91. Test-retest reliability ranges from .10 to .90, depending mostly on the time interval between test and retest.

Validity
Experimental validation studies in which particular Rorschach scores are tested with non-Rorschach criteria yield low coefficients in the range of .20 to .40. Recent studies have focused on clinical settings in which comparisons of Rorschach-based analyses and case-history-interview analyses were made. Resulting correlation coefficients ranged from −.20 to .74 with a mean of .37.

Norms
The Rorschach Method is not a psychometric test based on comparing an individual's score to a specific norm group. It is difficult to find much evidence of normative studies in the literature, except perhaps in the area of developmental changes related to age groups.

Norms for Hearing-Impaired People
None have been established.

Appropriateness for Hearing-Impaired People

The Rorschach Method has been used successfully with hearing-impaired people. Success in administration and valid results are primarily dependent on the evaluator's level of skill in communicating with hearing-impaired people. Because every detail of the interaction between the evaluator and client must be reported, total communication comprehension by both evaluator and client must be achieved.

Range of Scores

Scoring is a process of classification. Responses are put into categories and assigned a symbol. Researchers have developed various systems for classification and interpretation (Blum, 1954; Klopfer, 1954; Piotrowski, 1974). Responses are classified according to location (area of the blot used); determinant (those aspects of the blot that determine the concept); content score (description of concept, such as human, animal, hand-made object, etc.); and popularity or originality. A frequency count may be made of responses in each category; this can be expressed in terms of a percentage or ratio.

Interpretation

This is by far the most complex aspect of the Rorschach Method. To a large extent, interpretation depends on the scoring system the examiner is using and his/her training and clinical background. The types of responses and their frequencies are analyzed along with the relationships between them. Sequence analyses follow quantitative analyses. This consists of the examiner looking at the specific responses from a phenomenological perspective, attempting to get a holistic view of the individual. All of this information is used to describe the client's personality, usually in a report form.

Summary of Buros Institute Publications

According to the sixth edition of Buros's *Mental Measurements Yearbook* (pp. 478-509), the Rorschach Method is viewed as an instrument lacking reliability, validity, or acceptable use. The difference between the way the examiner writes his/her analysis and the way the recipient of the report understands it is emphasized. One reviewer recommends abandoning the Rorschach in clinical practice.

General References

Beck, S. J., & Molish, H. B. *Rorschach's test*. New York: Grune & Stratton, 1967.

Blum, L. *A Rorschach workbook*. New York: International Universities Press, 1954.

Klopfer, B., Ainsworth, M. A., Klopfer, W. G., & Hold, R. R. *Developments in the Rorschach technique*. New York: Harcourt, Brace and World, 1954.

Piotrowski, Z. A. *Perceptanalysis*. Philadelphia: Ex Libris, 1974.

References Related to Hearing-Impaired People

Altshuler, K. Z. Toward a psychology of deafness. *Journal of Communication Disorders*, 1978, *II*(2-3) 159-169.

Harris, F. *Language concepts and personality measurement in the deaf using the S-O Rorschach test*. Unpublished doctoral dissertation, Colorado State College, 1967.

Monroe, H. J. *A comparative Rorschach investigation of functional and non-functional hearing impairment*. Unpublished doctoral dissertation, University of Denver, 1957.

Talkington, L., & Reed, K. Rorschach response patterns of hearing-impaired retardates. *Perceptual and Motor Skills*, 1969, *29*(2), 546.

Tennessee Self Concept Scale

Author
W. H. Fitts

Publisher
Counselor Recordings and Tests
Box 6184
Acklen Station
Nashville, TN 37212

Price
$3.75 per specimen kit

Date of Edition
1965

General Purpose
The Tennessee Self Concept Scale (TSCS) is designed as a measure of self-concept for counseling, evaluation, or research purposes.

Description
The TSCS has 100 self-descriptive statements. The client circles one of five responses ranging from one (completely false) to five (completely true). There are two forms of the TSCS, a *counseling form* and a *clinical and research form*. The test booklet and answer sheet are the same for both forms; only the scoring and profiling systems are different. In the counseling form there are 14 profiled scores (one self-criticism score, nine self-esteem scores, three variability of response scores, and one distribution score). The clinical and research form includes the above plus 15 other profiled scores. Categories for these additional scores include defensive positive, general maladjustment, psychosis, personality disorder, neurosis, and personality integration.

Administration
The TSCS is self-administered and therefore may be given individually or to a group. Adequate instructions are provided in the test booklet; the publisher cautions that the answer sheet may be confusing as only every other item requires a response. The answer sheet, scoring sheet, and profile sheet are available in a combination packet in which marks on the answer sheet automatically register on the scoring and profile sheets. Total time required ranges from 10 to 20 minutes.

Special Administration Procedures for Hearing-Impaired People
No special administration procedures for hearing-impaired people have been established. The examiner may need to explain some word meanings; for this, fluency in sign language may be necessary.

Age Level
12 years and above (minimum reading level of sixth grade)

Reliability
The reliability coefficients for the TSCS range from .61 to .92. They were obtained from test-retest procedures using 60 college students over a two-week period.

Validity
Content validity was determined by unanimous agreement among seven clinical psychologists. Correlation coefficients with a few other personality measures were established. With the MMPI, correlation coefficients were satisfactory; with the Edwards Personal Preference Schedule, correlation coefficients were disappointingly low.

Norms
Norms were derived from a sample of 626 people ages 12 to 68 from various parts of the country. Individuals were both white and Black and had educational levels ranging from sixth grade to Ph.D. Individuals came from high school and college classes, employers at state institutions, and other sources. There was overrepresentation of college students, white individuals, and people between ages 12 and 30.

Norms for Hearing-Impaired People
No norms have been established.

Appropriateness for Hearing-Impaired People

For a postlingually deaf person, or for a hearing-impaired person with no language problems, the TSCS would be appropriate. Generally the test statements follow basic, simple syntax form. Interpretation of results requires an understanding of how hearing impairment affects self-concept.

Range of Scores

For both the counseling form and the clinical research form, raw scores are converted to percentiles and *T*-scores.

Interpretation

The counseling form gives 14 profiled scores which are useful for self-interpretation and for feedback to counselees. The clinical and research form includes all the counseling form scales plus 15 more. The clinical and research form is quite complex and therefore not appropriate for self-interpretation or counselee feedback; it is useful for research and diagnostic purposes, however.

Summary of Buros Institute Publications

Reviewed in the seventh edition of Buros's *Mental Measurements Yearbook* (Vol. 1, pp. 364-370). According to the reviewers the TSCS offers great potential as a promising clinical instrument. The empirical scales are useful as a means of screening clients for pathologies. The manual needs to be improved and there are some drawbacks related to the current scoring system.

General References

Wylie, R. C. *The self-concept* (Vol. 1: A review of methodological considerations and measuring instruments; Vol. 2: Theory and research on selected topics). Lincoln: University of Nebraska Press, 1979.

References Related to Hearing-Impaired People

Garrison, W. M., Tesch, S., & Decaro, P. An assessment of self-concept levels among post-secondary deaf adolescents. *American Annals of the Deaf*, 1978, *123*(8), 968-975.

Grey, G. *Identification, self-concept, and attitude toward disabled persons in selected groups of normal hearing and hearing-impaired adults.* Unpublished doctoral dissertation, Marquette University, 1976.

Sussman, A. *An investigation into the relationship between self concepts of deaf adults and their perceived attitudes toward deafness.* Unpublished doctoral dissertation, New York University, 1973.

Thematic Apperception Test

Author
H. A. Murray

Publisher
Harvard University Press
79 Garden Street
Cambridge, MA 02138

Price
$11.50 (cards and manual)

Date of Edition
1943

General Purpose
The Thematic Apperception Test (TAT) is designed as an investigative technique in which a trained clinical psychologist can interpret the dynamic, driving forces of one's personality. It helps the therapist to uncover the hidden complexities and conflicts of personality, drawing out emotions, sentiments, and desires manifested in the unconscious.

Description
The TAT consists of 19 black and white pictures printed on white bristol board, and one blank card. The examinee is instructed to make up a story as suggested by each picture card. The stories are recorded and interpreted at a later date.

Administration
The TAT may be administered individually or to a group, orally or written, and in one or more sessions. Murray (1951) recommends two sessions. Most people do not need any special preparation; for those individuals who have no educational or psychological testing experience, however, another less imposing test should be administered before taking the TAT. The examiner reads the instructions to the examinee. The examinee is given five minutes per picture card to speak or write a story. All verbal information is recorded by the examiner or a hidden stenographer. The total time required ranges from 45 to 60 minutes.

Special Administration Procedures for Hearing-Impaired People
No special administration procedures for hearing-impaired people have been established. Communication between evaluator and client is vital.

Age Level
4 years and above (but used primarily with adolescents and adults; a special version of the TAT—the Children's Apperception Test—is more appropriate for younger clients).

Reliability
Reliability data for the TAT are lacking due to the nature of the test and the changing moods of the examinee. Test-retest reliability is not high. However, Jensen, in his review of the test in the fifth edition of Buros's *Mental Measurements Yearbook* (p. 164), reported 15 estimates of scoring reliability ranging from .54 to .91. Jensen also revealed an average internal consistency reliability of .13. This would call for extreme caution.

Validity
Due to the changing moods of examinees, validity is still in question. However, Bellak (1954) reported on some early experiments which consisted of the examiner introducing post-hypnotic orders to feel aggressive. Thereafter, when the clients were instructed to provide stories of the same pictures, aggression was clearly projected. Split-half comparisons—between five stories told under these circumstances and five stories without induced aggression—showed that main personality characteristics persisted despite the artificial situation.

Norms
Not reported

Norms for Hearing-Impaired People
None have been established.

Appropriateness for Hearing-Impaired People

The TAT can be used with a hearing-impaired person if the examiner and the examinee have a common, fluent method of communication. In some cases this means that the examiner would need a full and comprehensive understanding of American Sign Language (ASL), because the examiner is required to record verbatim everything the examinee says. Videotaping of responses has been attempted with hearing-impaired people. The advantage of videotape is that interpretation could be made at a later date by a person who fully understands ASL. The disadvantage of this approach is that the spontaneity of questions and answers between examiner and client at the time of testing would be lost. Because of varied English-language levels and usage, writing of stories by hearing-impaired people is not recommended.

Range of Scores

The TAT is not based on the comparison of scores with standard norms. Norms are subjective, based on the author's clinical experience with the test. Murray (1951) bases scores on identification of "needs" and "presses." A "need" is equivalent to an attribute of the hero representing tendencies in the examinee's personality. These tendencies belong to the person's past or anticipated future. A "press" represents forces in the individual's environment, past, present, or future. A list of need variables is identified. Then a range of scores from one to five is used to rate each need variable. A rating of five is the highest possible score for any variable in a single story. After the 20 stories have been scored with reference to intensity, duration, frequency, and importance in the plot, the total for each variable is compared with a standard score (if available) for examinees of the given age and sex. Scores that vary above and below the standards are listed and scrutinized in relation to each other.

Interpretation

Before interpreting the test, the examiner should know the sex and age of the examinee, whether his/her parents are dead or separated, the age and sex of all siblings, and the person's vocation and marital status. The TAT has been interpreted in many ways. Bellak (1954) outlined several procedures: (1) the simplest procedure is the inspection technique, whereby the examiner rereads the stories, looking for patterns and how the patterns fit a meaningful whole; (2) in psychotherapy the examinee and therapist hold carbon copies of the stories, and the examinee is invited to freely associate and interpret the stories; and (3) Murray (1951) utilized the need-press method, whereby every sentence was analyzed as to the needs of the hero, and the environmental forces (press) to which the client is exposed (see Range of Scores).

Summary of Buros Institute Publications

Discussed in the sixth edition of Buros's *Mental Measurements Yearbook* (pp. 244-246). The reviewers are highly critical of reliability and validity. In the hands of a qualified and experienced examiner, however, the TAT can be a useful tool in psychotherapy. The reviewers recommend that further testing be done.

General References

Bellak, L. *The Thematic Apperception Test and the Children's Apperception Test in clincial use.* New York: Grune & Stratton, 1954.

Christenson, J. A., Jr. Clinical application of the Thematic Apperception Test. *Journal of Abnormal and Social Psychology*, 1943, *38*, 104-106.

Murray, H. A. Uses of the TAT. *American Journal of Psychiatry*, 1951, *107*, 577-581.

Rapaport, D., Gill, M., & Schafer, R. *Diagnostic psychological testing.* New York: International Universities Press, 1968.

Tomkins, S.S. The limits of material obtainable in a single case study by daily administration of the Thematic Apperception Test. *Psychological Bulletin*, 1942, *39*, 490.

References Related to Hearing-Impaired People

None available

5 VISUAL PERCEPTION TESTS

BENDER VISUAL-MOTOR GESTALT TEST FOR YOUNG CHILDREN
Koppitz Scoring System

Author
L. Bender and E. M. Koppitz

Publisher
Grune & Stratton, Inc.
111 Fifth Avenue
New York, NY 10003

Price
$20.50 per set (manual and cards)
$12.75 per package (25 scoring sheets)

Date of Edition
1963

General Purpose
The Bender Visual-Motor Gestalt Test is used to determine the process of maturation of visual motor perception in young children. It is also used to determine school readiness, predict school achievement, diagnose problems in reading and arithmetic, diagnose brain injury, determine the degree of mental retardation, and evaluate emotional disturbances in young children.

Description
The test consists of nine figures on separate cards which are presented to the child one at a time. The child is then asked to copy each figure on a blank piece of paper.

Administration
The test is designed to be administered individually. Blank sheets of 8½ by 11 paper and a No. 2 pencil must be supplied. The paper is placed in front of the child in a vertical position. The examiner then issues the instructions: "I have nine cards here with designs on them for you to copy. Here is the first one. Now go ahead and make one like it." Each child is permitted to use as much or as little paper as he/she desires. The test does not have any time limit. Total time required ranges from 10 to 20 minutes.

Special Administration Procedures for Hearing-Impaired People

No special administration procedures for hearing-impaired people have been established. Because the instructions are simple, they may be easily pantomimed or demonstrated. A minimum of verbal communication is necessary.

Age Level

5 to 10 years

Reliability

Two aspects of the Koppitz Scoring System must be considered in order to demonstrate its reliability: scorer reliability, that is, the agreement among different scorers independently using the scoring system; and test score reliability, that is, the consistency of the test scores for subjects to whom the test has been administered more than once. For scorer reliability, correlations ranged from .88 to .96. For test score reliability, a test-retest method (with a four-month interval) produced a reliability coefficient of .61.

Validity

Chi-squares were computed comparing individuals, with and without learning problems, whose Bender scores were above or below the mean score for their particular grade level. All three chi-squares were statistically significant at the .01 level. Little information on validity of the Bender test is available, according to the sixth and seventh editions of Buros's *Mental Measurements Yearbook*. Koppitz (1975) presents high validities in evaluating school readiness and success in the first grade. Data also indicate that the Koppitz Scoring System has good validity with mentally retarded children in terms of subsequent school achievement.

Norms

Normative data were derived from 1,104 public school children representing 46 classes in 12 different schools located in rural, small town, suburban, and urban areas of the Midwest and East. All of the children were above 5 and below 11 years old.

Norms for Hearing-Impaired People

Research indicates no significant difference on scores for the hearing-impaired children based on the hearing impairment alone (Levine, 1974).

Appropriateness for Hearing-Impaired People

This test is used widely with hearing-impaired children. The instructions for the test are very simple and easily pantomimed, if necessary. In addition, sign language, the manual alphabet, or any other nonverbal mode of communication may be used to clarify the task requested of the child. Most importantly, the test is a performance test rather than a verbal test. One note of caution: Children with visual acuity problems and/or manual dexterity problems should not be given this test; hearing-impaired children should be screened for these possible problems before administration of this test.

Range of Scores

Using the Koppitz Scoring System, the Bender test is scored for errors. A high score indicates a poor performance; a low score reflects a good performance. There are 31 scoring items in the Koppitz system. For children age 10, the mean score is 1.5 with a standard deviation of 2.10. For children 5 years old, the mean score is 13.6 with a standard deviation of 3.61.

Interpretation

A child's score on the Koppitz Scoring System can be compared with other children (1) of the same chronological age, (2) with the same level of maturation in visual-motor perception, and (3) at a given grade level. No specific classification system is used.

Summary of Buros Institute Publications

Discussed in the seventh edition of Buros's *Mental Measurements Yearbook* (Vol. 1, pp. 390-395). The Bender test should be included in every diagnostic examination of children because of its unique contribution to the evaluation of perceptual-motor functioning. Koppitz's scoring system and scoring manual provide useful aids in application of the Bender to the study of children's problems.

General References

Baldwin, M. V. A note regarding the suggested use of the Bender Gestalt Test as a measure of school readiness. *Journal of Clinical Psychology*, 1950, *6*, 412.

Connor, J. P. Bender Gestalt Test performance as a predictor of differential reading performance. *Journal of School Psychology*, 1968-69, *7*, 41-44.

Koppitz, E. M. The Bender Gestalt Test and learning disturbances in young children. *Journal of Clinical Psychology*, 1958, *14*, 292-295.

References Related to Hearing-Impaired People

Clarke, B. R., & Leslie, P. T. Visual-motor skills and reading ability of deaf children. *Perceptual and Motor Skills*, 1971, *33*(1), 263-269.

Gilbert, J., & Levee, R. T. Performances of deaf and normally hearing children educationally designated as brain damaged. *American Journal of Orthopsychiatry*, 1969, *39*, 437-446.

Levine, E. S. Psychological tests and practices with the deaf: A survey. *Volta Review*, 1974, *76*, 298-319.

Master, I. *Bender Gestalt responses of normal and deaf children.* Unpublished master's thesis, Brooklyn College, 1962.

Myklebust, H. R., & Brutten, M. A study of the visual perception of deaf children. *ACTA Otolaryngological Supplement*, 1963, *105*, 1-126.

BENTON VISUAL RETENTION TEST

Author
A. L. Benton

Publisher
The Psychological Corporation
757 Third Avenue
New York, NY 10017

Price
$12.75 (manual, design cards, and 50 scoring sheets)

Date of Edition
1955

General Purpose
The Benton Visual Retention Test (BVRT) is a clinical and research instrument designed to assess memory, perception, and visual-motor reproductions. The BVRT is designed to provide a diagnostic assessment of organic brain disorder in children and adults.

Description
The BVRT consists of three equivalent forms: C, D, and E. In each form there are ten designs; each design consists of one or more geometric figures. The client is told to draw the figure(s), recreating the original design as much as possible.

Administration
The BVRT is designed to be administered individually. The client is given a blank sheet of paper, the same size as the cards on which the test material is printed, and a pencil with an eraser. There are four methods of presenting the BVRT. In administration A, the 10 designs of a given form are presented to the individual at an exposure rate of 10 seconds per design. In administration B, the exposure is five seconds. The design remains in view of the individual for administration C. For administration D, the exposure is 10 seconds then a 15 second delay before response is permitted. Designs should be positioned at an angle of about 60 degrees to permit

optimal viewing. Individuals are permitted to make erasures or corrections. No spontaneous praise is to be given by the examiner. Regardless of form, total time required ranges from 10 to 20 minutes.

Special Administration Procedures for Hearing-Impaired People

No special administration procedures for hearing-impaired people have been established. The performance nature of the administration of the BVRT, however, lends itself to using this test with hearing-impaired people.

Age Level

6 years, 6 months and above

Reliability

Test-retest reliablities for administration A, estimated by the correlation coefficient among alternate forms, was found to be approximately .85. Comparing alternate Forms C and D with a group of 35 adults, the author found a mean correct score of 6.4 for Form C and 5.7 for Form D.

Validity

Concurrent validation was obtained through a study of 34 neuropsychiatric patients. Correlations were assessed from patients' performance on the BVRT compared with electroencephalograph findings. Eighty-three percent of the patients with EEG abnormalities showed defective performance on the BVRT. Correlation between the BVRT and the WAIS were found to be positive with correlations of .61 for full-scale IQ, .61 for verbal IQ, and .52 for performance IQ. The median correlation with the WAIS subtests was .60.

Norms

Normative data for the BVRT have been established for the three forms. Though designed for equal difficulty, studies have shown Form C (using administration A) is slightly easier than Forms D and E. Norms for administration C (copying for design) were derived separately for adults and children. The adult control group consisted of 200 medical patients with no history of cerebral disease. The study group consisted of 100 patients with diagnosed cerebral disease. Children's norms for administration C were derived from the performance of 236 children between ages 6 years, 6 months and 13 years, 5 months enrolled in public schools in Iowa and Wisconsin. The norm group was randomly selected with the sole criterion that WISC-R full-scale IQs be between 85 and 115. The mean WISC-R full-scale IQ of the norm group was 102.5.

Norms for Hearing-Impaired People

None have been established.

Appropriateness for Hearing-Impaired People

The BVRT has been used with hearing-impaired people. Since the BVRT is nonverbal, administration procedures can be demonstrated easily through example. Use of existing normative data would appear appropriate.

Range of Scores

Two scoring systems are available for the evaulation of individual performance. One score of correct reproductions provides a measure of general efficiency of performance. The second type is an error score, which measures specific kinds of errors. The range of possible error and correct scores for any single form of the test is 0 to 10. Errors are similar to other tests of visual-motor perception, that is, distortions, perseverations, rotations, omissions, misplacements, and size errors. The author noted no significant improvement in correct scores after examinees reach age 13.

Interpretation

The BVRT scores which fall below the expected level are clinically significant. The manual contains cut-off scores for both children and adults by age groups. The perceptual component of the BVRT (copying for design) is associated with functioning of the right parieto-occipital region of the brain. In a study of 100 right-side-brain-injured adults and 100 control cases, Benton (1962, 1964) found that a score of three points below expected number of correct drawings correctly identified 57 percent of the brain-damaged patients. The author suggests that this test not be used as the sole criterion for diagnosis.

Summary of Buros Institute Publications

Discussed in the fifth edition of Buros's *Mental Measurements Yearbook* (pp. 535-537). The reviewers state that, while the BVRT claims to be a clinical instrument designed to assess memory and perception, in reality the test is one of memory for design, not memory in general. The BVRT does not separate perceptual factors from memory factors except in administration C, which does not measure memory. Important data are absent from the test manual, including statistical methods, reliability, and correlations among the alternate forms of the test. The test is still in an experimental stage.

General References

Benton, A. L. Visual Retention Test as a constructional praxis task. *Confinia Nuerologia*, 1962, *22*, 141-155.

Benton, A. L., & Spreen, O. Visual memory test performance in mentally deficient and brain damaged patients. *American Journal of Mental Deficiency*, 1964, *68*, 630-633.

Benton, A. L., Spreen, O., Fangman, M., & Carr, D. L. Visual Retention Test administration C: Norms for children. *Journal of Special Education*, 1967, *1*(2), 151-156.

Lacks, P. Revised interpretation of Benton Visual Retention Test scores. *Journal of Clinical Psychology*, 1971, *27*, 481-482.

References Related to Hearing-Impaired People

Goetzinger, C. P., & Huber, T. G. A study of immediate and delayed visual retention with deaf and hearing adolescents. *American Annals of the Deaf*, 1964, *109*, 297-305.

MEMORY FOR DESIGNS TEST

Author
F. K. Graham and B. S. Kendall

Publisher
Psychological Tests Specialists
Box 9229
Missoula, MT 59801

Price
$8.50 (test materials and manual)

Date of Edition
1960

General Purpose
The Memory for Designs Test (MFD) is designed as a test of visual memory used to identify organic brain disorders.

Description
The test materials consist of 15 five-inch cardboard squares with a geometric design printed in black on each square.

Administration
The MFD is designed to be administered individually. The individual is given a pencil with an eraser and an 8½ by 11 sheet of blank white paper. The examiner explains to the individual that each card will be presented for five seconds and that the person is then expected to reproduce each design. The examiner may remind the person not to start drawing until the card is removed. Total time required is 15 minutes.

Special Administration Procedures for Hearing-Impaired People
No special administration procedures for hearing-impaired people have been established. The performance nature of the items lends itself to use with hearing-impaired people.

Age Level
8 years, 5 months and above

Reliability

Immediate test-retest reliabilities are reported in the range of .72 to .90. Retesting after 10-day intervals indicated that patients with cortical brain damage show a higher practice effort than do schizophrenics.

Validity

Validity reportedly varies widely depending on the type of sample group used. In studies of matched validation and cross-validation groups, the correct identification of brain-damaged patients varied between 42 and 50 percent. Other studies report correct classifications ranging from 63 to 90 percent of brain-damaged patients. The predictive validity of the MFD correlates at a .001 significance level with the Bender Gestalt Test and the Benton Visual Retention Test. Studies of predictive validity suggest that the MFD is of more value in the diagnosis of severely brain-damaged patients than in the diagnosis of mildly impaired patients.

Norms

Norms are based on the performance of matched validation groups: a control group of 70 people including neurotics and psychotics, and a brain-damaged group of the same number. Both groups had an age range from 8 years, 6 months to 60 years.

Norms for Hearing-Impaired People

None have been established.

Appropriateness for Hearing-Impaired People

It appears that the MFD may be administered through sign language or gesture without upsetting standard administration procedures. Because the test requires no reading or verbal skills, it appears to be appropriate for most hearing-impaired people. Hearing-impaired people who have visual acuity or manual dexterity problems should not be given this test. Screening procedures should be implemented.

Range of Scores

The MFD raw scores range from 0 to 28. The score for each design is determined by the number and kind of errors made; the higher the score, the poorer the performance. The complex scoring system is included in the manual. It includes a chart for determining a differential score which statistically controls for the effects of chronological age and vocabulary level. The mean score of the matched control group was 3.47 with a standard deviation of 4.62. The mean score for the brain-damaged group was 11.54 with a standard deviation of 7.3.

Interpretation

The interpretation of raw scores for adults is by classification: 0 to 4 indicates "normal," 5 to 11 indicates "borderline," and 12 and above indicates "brain damage." Predicted raw scores based on chronological age and on intelligence measures are also provided.

Summary of Buros Institute Publications

As discussed in the sixth edition of Buros's *Mental Measurements Yearbook* (pp. 296-298), the MFD is more appropriate for diagnosis of severely brain-damaged people than of mildly impaired people. Improvements in the scoring system are suggested. A re-evaluation of the necessity for age corrections, and the possible refinement in the scoring of qualitative errors in relation to locus of lesion, may increase the usefulness of the MFD.

General References

May, A. E., Urquhart, A., & Watts, R. E. Memory for Designs Test: A follow-up study. *Perceptual and Motor Skills*, 1970, *30*, 753-754.

McManis, D. L. Memory for Designs performance of brain damaged and nonbrain damaged psychiatric patients. *Perceptual and Motor Skills*, 1974, *38*, 847-852.

References Related to Hearing-Impaired People

Clarke, B. R., & Leslie, P. T. Visual-motor skills and reading ability of deaf children. *Perceptual and Motor Skills*, 1971, *33*(1), 263-268.

MOTOR-FREE VISUAL PERCEPTION TEST

Author
R. P. Colarusso and D. D. Hammill

Publisher
Academic Therapy Publications
20 Commercial Boulevard
Novato, CA 94947

Price
$5.60 (50 scoring sheets)
$8.00 (manual)
$18.00 (test plates)

Date of Edition
1972

General Purpose
The Motor-Free Visual Perception Test (MVPT) is designed as a test of visual perception which avoids motor involvement. It is used for screening, diagnostic, and research purposes by teachers, psychologists, educational specialists, and others.

Description
The MVPT is a 36-item test with multiple choice responses. Test items are grouped according to five perceptual categories: *spatial relationship, visual discrimination, figure-ground, visual closure,* and *visual memory.* Test items within each category are arranged in order of difficulty. The test items consist of geometric shapes, letter-like and number-like forms, stick figures, and realistic designs.

Administration
The MVPT is designed to be administered individually. Each section has its own specific administration directions. A sample item for each section is provided to ensure that the child understands the directions. The only response required from the child is that he/she point to one of the four alternatives. The child is not allowed to trace any figures. The examiner should encourage the person to look at all four alternatives before making a final decision. The test is not timed; the child should be given a reasonable amount of time to make each selection. Total time required ranges from 15 to 30 minutes.

Special Administration Procedures for Hearing-Impaired People
No special administration procedures for hearing-impaired people have been established. Repetition of the instructions is encouraged.

Age Level
4 to 8 years

Reliability
Three reliability procedures—test-retest, split-half, and Kuder-Richardson—were performed on the MVPT. Due to the objective scoring procedures, inter-scorer reliability was not investigated. A reliability coefficient of .81 was derived from the scores of 162 children, selected from the standardization population, who were retested 20 days after pretesting. A reliability coefficient of .88 was found from the scores of the entire standardization population (881) using split-half reliability procedures. A reliability coefficient of .86 was determined from the scores of the entire standardization population using the Kuder-Richardson reliability procedures.

Validity
Content validity was checked by examining the test content to determine whether all aspects of visual perception were included in the MVPT. A correlation of .73 was found between the MVPT and the Frostig Test of Visual Perception.

Norms
The MVPT was standardized on a sample of 881 "normal" children ages 4 to 8 who resided in 22 states. Children identified as mentally retarded or sensorially handicapped were excluded. The data pool included samples from all races, economic levels, and residential areas. Differences between sexes and geographic areas were pooled for the purpose of determining norms.

Norms for Hearing-Impaired People
None have been established.

Appropriateness for Hearing-Impaired People

The test appears appropriate for administration to hearing-impaired people. It involves no language or speech skills. Demonstration and repetition of instructions may be used. Visual acuity should be tested before administration of this test.

Range of Scores

The MVPT raw scores range from 0 to 36. Perceptual ages for each raw score are then established by the mean test-age method (Table 7 in the test manual). Perceptual quotients are derived from the mean and standard deviation of raw scores associated with each six-month age interval (Table 9 in the manual). The mean perceptual quotient is 100 with a standard deviation of 15.

Interpretation

According to the author, only those raw scores of 10 or above can be interpreted with confidence. Lower scores indicate less than chance performance.

Summary of Buros Institute Publications

Discussed in the eighth edition of Buros's *Mental Measurements Yearbook* (Vol. 2, pp. 1417–1419). According to one reviewer, this test claims to be a quick, practical screening and diagnostic instrument, but inadequate evidence is presented to substantiate its validity for either screening or diagnosis. Consequently, the MVPT cannot be recommended in its present state. A second reviewer disagrees, calling the MVPT a quick, highly reliable, and valid measure of over-all visual perceptual processing ability.

General References

Hammill, D. Training visual perceptual processes. *The Journal of Learning Disabilities*, 1972, *5*, 552–559.

Hammill, D., & Bartel, N. *Teaching children with learning and behavior problems*. Boston: Allyn and Bacon, 1975.

Newcomer, P., & Hammill, D. Visual perception of motor impaired children: Implications for assessment. *Exceptional Children*, 1973, *39*, 335–336.

References Related to Hearing-Impaired People

None available

REITAN-INDIANA NEUROPSYCHOLOGICAL TEST BATTERY FOR CHILDREN

Author

R. M. Reitan

Publisher

Neuropsychological Laboratory
1338 Edison Street
Tucson, AZ 85719

Date of Edition

1979

Price

$950.00 (testing equipment)
$32.00 (forms)

General Purpose

The Reitan-Indiana Neuropsychological Test Battery for Children (R-INT) is a test of organic functioning. It is designed to provide complete and definitive results in the assessment of brain damage, particularly lesion sites and their effects on behavior.

Description

The R-INT is a modification of the batteries designed by Halstead and Reitan for older children and adults. The R-INT consists of subtests covering the following skills and traits: visual-spatial relationships, simple abstraction or concept formation, organizational ability, flexibility in thinking, motor-speed, sensory-perception, immediate alertness, and incidental memory. The R-INT is always given in conjunction with the Aphasia Screening Battery, Sensory-Perceptual Examination, and appropriate Wechsler intelligence scales.

Administration

The R-INT is designed to be administered individually. The administration is complex and time consuming, usually taking a full day and sometimes longer. The manual provides thorough instructions for each subtest, and practice sheets are used for many of them. Examiners are strongly advised not to administer this test without specific training. According to the author, administering the test and interpreting the results requires extensive knowledge and experience in clinical neuropsychology and psychoanalysis.

Special Administration Procedures for Hearing-Impaired People

No special administration procedures for hearing-impaired people have been established.

Age Level

5 to 8 years

Reliability

The manual provides no information on reliability. Other researchers have tested the reliability of other batteries in the Halstead-Reitan group. Matarazzo, Wiens, Matarazzo, and Goldstein (1974) found the reliability of the R-INT satisfactory in identifying "normal" and afflicted individuals for an older age group.

Validity

There is no mention of validity in the manual, and no other statistics are available for this particular battery. In 1955, however, Reitan did cross-validation studies of the earlier forms of Halstead's batteries, differentiating between clients with brain damage and those without. Through further research, Vega and Parsons (1967) verified Reitan's results. Filskov and Goldstein (1974) demonstrated that, in determining location of lesions and the psychological process affected, the R-INT had a higher "hit rate" (identifying known cases) than a brain scan, electroencephalogram, angiogram, pneumoencephalogram, and x-ray.

Norms

Not provided

Norms for Hearing-Impaired People

None have been established.

Appropriateness for Hearing-Impaired People

Many of the subtests of the batteries for older age groups are highly verbal and therefore inappropriate for a majority of hearing-impaired people. Most of these subtests have been eliminated for the younger age group's battery. Test interpretation depends more on the knowledge and experience of the examiner than on specific numerical scores. Therefore, an examiner with the background necessary to account for clients' hearing losses and other related physiological and psychological conditions could make good use of this test with hearing-impaired people. Research is needed on the appropriateness of the R-INT for hearing-impaired people.

Range of Scores

Each subtest has a separate scoring system, with most scores recorded in raw score/number of errors.

Interpretation

Results of tests are given in terms of lesion sites suspected, if any, and their effects on psychological functioning and behavior. Recommendations for therapy or educational placement follow from the results.

Summary of Buros Institute Publications

The R-INT is not reviewed in Buros's *Mental Measurements Yearbooks*.

General References

Filskov, S. B., & Goldstein, S. G. Diagnostic validity of the Halstead-Reitan neuropsychological battery. *Journal of Consulting and Clinical Psychology*, 1974, 42(3), 382–388.

Maloney, M., & Ward, M. *Psychological assessment: A conceptual approach.* New York: Oxford University Press, 1976.

Matarazzo, J. D., Wiens, A. N., Matarazzo, R. G., & Goldstein, S. C. Psychometric and clinical test-retest reliability of the Halstead impairment index in a sample of healthy, young normal men. *Journal of Nervous and Mental Disease,* 1974, *158,* 37–49.

Reitan, R., & Davidson, L. (Eds.). *Clinical neuropsychology: Current status and applications.* Washington, D. C.: V. H. Winston & Sons, 1974.

Scott, A., Williams, J., & Stout, J. Review of the literature on learning disabilities. In J. Szuhay & B. Newhill (Project Directors), *Field investigation and evaluation of learning disabilities* (Vol. 1). Scranton: University of Scranton Press, 1980.

Vega, A. J., & Parsons, O. A. Cross validation of the Halstead-Reitan tests for brain damage. *Journal of Consulting Psychology,* 1967, *31*(6), 619–625.

References Related to Hearing-Impaired People

None available

6
VOCATIONAL APTITUDE TESTS

BENNETT MECHANICAL COMPREHENSION TESTS

Author
G. K. Bennett

Publisher
The Psychological Corporation
757 Third Avenue
New York, NY 10017

Price
$13.50 (package of 25 tests)
$1.65 (manual)
$1.65 (key)
$6.25 (package of 25 answer sheets)

Date of Edition
1970

General Purpose
The Bennett Mechanical Comprehension Tests (BMCT) is designed to measure the ability to perceive and understand the relationship of physical forces and mechanical elements in practical situations.

Description
The BMCT is a revision of Tests of Mechanical Comprehension. The BMCT is suitable for applicants for industrial and mechanical jobs, high school students interested in such jobs, and candidates for engineering schools.

There are two parallel forms of the BMCT, Forms S and T. The reading level for both forms is in the "fairly easy" range, similar to that used in popular magazines. Each form is in a reusable booklet. The test consists of 68 questions accompanied by large, clear illustrations of mechanisms and contrivances. The individual is asked to use a separate answer sheet.

Administration

The BMCT may be administered individually or in a group. Instructions are usually given orally; the individual reads each question to himself/herself. The examination may also be administered by tape for those with limited reading ability. Both forms are timed tests with 30-minute limits.

Special Administration Procedures for Hearing-Impaired People

No special administration procedures for hearing-impaired people have been established. The format of the test is inappropriate for hearing-impaired people who cannot fully comprehend the written instructions and written test items.

Age Level

Grades 9 to 12 and adults

Reliability

Reliability coefficients are based on split-half correlations with the coefficients corrected for the full length of the test by the Spearman-Brown formula. The range of reliability coefficients vary from .81 to .93 with a median of .86. The standard errors of measurement range from 3.0 to 3.8.

Validity

In contrast to earlier forms of BMCT (Forms AA and BB), there has been relatively little validity testing done on Forms S and T. There are five validity coefficients available ranging from .12 to .52 with a median of .24. The criteria used as measures of validity are shop grades, job ratings, performance ratings, quality of work, and course grades in science.

Norms

Norms are presented for industrial applicants, industrial employees, and students (grades 11 and 12 in academic or technical high school). The mean score for industrial employees was 55.5. The mean for industrial applicants ranged from 43.3 to 47.5. The mean scores for academic high school students were 36.9 (grade 11) and 37.4 (grade 12). Technical high school scores were somewhat higher than academic high school scores, with mean scores of 40.6 (grade 11) and 42.2 (grade 12).

Norms for Hearing-Impaired People

None have been established.

Appropriateness for Hearing-Impaired People

The BMCT is written at approximately a sixth-grade reading level, which may be too difficult for some hearing-impaired people. Several of the test questions are inappropriate for hearing-impaired people because they relate to sound.

Range of Scores

Raw scores are converted to percentiles for various norm groups by using tables in the manual.

Interpretation

A counselor may compare a person's raw score with the tables of norm groups to see if the person compares favorably, for example, with industrial employees.

Summary of Buros Institute Publications

Discussed in the seventh edition of Buros's *Mental Measurements Yearbook* (Vol. 2, pp. 1483-1487). The reviews are varied, with one reviewer stating that the test is of limited value and that evidence of its predictive usefulness is very inadequate; another reviewer calls the BMCT "an energetic revision" of the earlier forms and states that the test has "a new lease on life."

General References

Cass, J. C., & Tiedeman, D. V. Vocational development and the election of a high school curriculum. *Personnel and Guidance Journal*, 1960, *38*, 538-545.

Crane, W. J. Screening devices for occupational therapy majors. *American Journal of Occupational Therapy*, 1962, *16*, 131-132.

Owens, W. A. A comment on the recent study of the Mechanical Comprehension Test (CC) by R. L. Decker. *Journal of Applied Psychology*, 1959, *43*, 31.

References Related to Hearing-Impaired People

None available

DIFFERENTIAL APTITUDE TESTS

Author
G. K. Bennett, H. G. Seashore, and A. G. Wesman

Publisher
The Psychological Corporation
757 Third Avenue
New York, NY 10017

Price
$32.00 (package of 25 tests)

Date of Edition
1975

General Purpose
The original Differential Aptitude Tests (DAT) was developed in 1947 to provide an integrated, scientific, and well-standardized procedure for measuring the abilities of boys and girls in grades 8 through 12 for purposes of educational and vocational counseling. The DAT was revised and restandardized in 1962 (Forms L and M) and again in 1975 (Forms S and T). Two new forms in 1981 (Forms V and W) will not be reviewed here.

Description
There are eight subtests of the DAT: *verbal reasoning, numerical ability, abstract reasoning, clerical speed and accuracy, mechanical reasoning, space relations, language usage I—spelling,* and *language usage II—grammar.* The verbal reasoning, numerical ability, and abstract reasoning subtests measure those functions which are associated with general ability, that is, scholastic aptitude or intelligence. Mechanical reasoning and space relations relate to a student's ability to recognize everyday physical forces and principles, and to visualize concrete objects and manipulate those visualizations. The clerical speed and accuracy, spelling, and language usage subtests are designed to assess skills necessary for various levels of office work.

Administration
The DAT may be administered individually or to a group. Forms S and T, each with eight subtests, are contained in separate booklets. Answers are marked on separate answer sheets which can be scored either by hand or machine. All subtests should be given within a one- to two-week period. Testing can be divided into two, four, or six sessions. The examiner may present the directions for each subtest orally but is not allowed to give different explanations or examples. The total time required for each form is 4 hours.

Special Administration Procedures for Hearing-Impaired People
No special administration procedures for hearing-impaired people have been established. Repetition of the instructions is encouraged. Alteration of instructions is not encouraged.

Age Level
Grades 8 through 12

Reliability
At each grade level, reliability coefficients for each of the subtests were computed separately for males and females with both forms, S and T. The reliability coefficients were computed by correlating raw scores of odd- and even-numbered items for all subtests (except the clerical speed and accuracy subtest, which was done by an alternate form method). Each of these reliability samples included approximately 250 people. Reliability coefficients ranged from .78 to .97. Forms S and T have generally higher reliability coefficients than the old forms; the standard errors of measurement are approximately the same for the new and old forms.

Validity
The amount of validity data available on the DAT is overwhelming, including several thousand validity coefficients. Most of the data concerns predictive validity in terms of high school achievement and, to a more limited extent, college achievement. Correlation coefficients are reported between separate course-grade criteria and each of the DAT tests. Validity coefficients were computed separately for males, females, and grade levels. Validity coefficients varied among subtests, ranging from .19 to .70.

Norms

The norms for Forms S and T are based on more than 64,000 students in grades 8 through 12 at 76 public and parochial schools throughout the United States. In general, for any grade-sex-form group, the same sample weight was applied to cases from all school districts within a sampling unit. In some areas, however, the estimated proportion of Black students tested was in excess of the expected figures.

Norms for Hearing-Impaired People

None have been established.

Appropriateness for Hearing-Impaired People

The verbal nature of many of the subtests as well as the administration procedures make this test inappropriate for many hearing-impaired people. Extreme caution should be used in interpreting the results, especially results related to verbal subtests.

Range of Scores

Raw scores are converted to percentiles and stanines. Percentile rankings applicable to Forms S and T are presented separately for each grade and sex.

Interpretation

Percentile scores of the DAT can assist the counselor with client decisions of educational and vocational planning, training, and placement.

Summary of Buros Institute Publications

Discussed in the eighth edition of Buros's *Mental Measurements Yearbook* (Vol. 1, pp. 654–665). Reviewers' criticisms of Forms S and T are related to the heavy male orientation of the mechanical reasoning and the two language usage subtests. Evidence suggests that the DAT achieves very little differential validity and primarily measures general intelligence. All scales show excellent reliability. Women are under-represented in the tests. Blacks are over-represented.

General References

Bennett, G. K., Seashore, H. G., & Wesman, A. G. *Fifth edition manual for the Differential Aptitude Tests, Forms S & T.* New York: The Psychological Corporation, 1974.

Doppelt, J. E., & Seashore, H. G. How effective are your tests? *Test Service Bulletin* (No. 37). New York: The Psychological Corporation, June 1949.

Elton, C. F., & Morris, D. The use of the DAT in a small liberal arts college. *Journal of Educational Research*, 1956, *50*, 139–143.

References Related to Hearing-Impaired People

None available

Flanagan Industrial Tests

Author
J. Flanagan

Publisher
Science Research Associates, Inc.
1540 Page Mill Road
Palo Alto, CA 94304

Price
$9.45 (package of 25 tests)
$3.80 (scoring stencil)
$2.60 (manual)
$12.90 (specimen set)

Date of Edition
1960

General Purpose
The Flanagan Industrial Tests (FIT) is a general vocational aptitude battery designed for use in personnel selection and placement programs for a wide variety of jobs.

Description
The FIT is composed of 18 subtests: arithmetic, assembly, components, coordination, electronics, expression, ingenuity, inspection, judgement and comprehension, mathematics and reasoning, mechanics, memory, patterns, planning, precision, scales, tables, and vocabulary.

Administration
The FIT is designed to be administered individually. The directions for administering all tests assume that the examinee has at least some literacy and test-taking skills. Modification of the recommended procedure will be required if the tests are administered to educationally disadvantaged applicants. Not all 18 subtests need be administered; subtests can be selected as appropriate for a particular job or jobs being considered. Total administration time for all 18 subtests is 3½ hours.

Special Administration Procedures for Hearing-Impaired People
No special administration procedures for hearing-impaired people have been established.

Age Level
High school graduates and above

Reliability
Only indirect evidence of reliability is available. Correlations were obtained between the FIT and the Flanagan Aptitude Classification Test batteries administered to several high school and college groups. Correlations were all below .80; for eight of the subtests, they were in the .50s.

Validity
No information available

Norms
Norms are based on a sample of 3,359 twelfth-grade students and a sample of 701 first-year students entering a selected university. Neither of these samples would appear to be representative of the adults encountered in personnel selection programs for a wide variety of jobs.

Norms for Hearing-Impaired People
None have been established.

Appropriateness for Hearing-Impaired People
Because the FIT is a paper-and-pencil test requiring reading skills, and because no norms have been established for a hearing-impaired population, this test would not seem appropriate for most hearing-impaired people.

Range of Scores
Raw scores can be converted to percentiles and stanines for comparison purposes with industrial and business personnel, twelfth-grade students, and entering first-year college students.

Interpretation

Effective use of the FIT depends on knowing what requirements are important for successful job performance. For most jobs, a personnel manager can select four to eight subtests and obtain a composite score that reflects an individual's qualifications regarding that job.

Summary of Buros Institute Publications

Discussed in the seventh edition of Buros's *Mental Measurements Yearbook* (Vol. 2, pp. 1377-1382). The reviewers conclude that the FIT is a useful addition to tools available for vocational guidance. More validity and reliability data should be collected. At present, the test seems well-suited for research in personnel selection.

General References

Penfield, R. V. *The psychological characteristics of effective first line managers.* Unpublished doctoral dissertation, Cornell University, 1966.

References Related to Hearing-Impaired People

None available

GENERAL APTITUDE TEST BATTERY

Author

U. S. Employment Service

Publisher

Specialty Case Manufacturing Co.
Test Equipment Inc.
P. O. Box 495
Huntingdon Valley, PA 19006

Price

$40.80 (manual, test forms, and scoring apparatus)
$31.00 (pegboard and finger dexterity apparatus)
$3.60 (100 hand-processing score cards)

Date of Edition

1979

General Purpose

The General Aptitude Test Battery (GATB) is a multiple aptitude test battery designed to measure capacities to learn various jobs. Nine aptitudes are matched to 66 different job clusters. These clusters cover nonsupervisory occupations.

Description

The GATB consists of 12 subtests: name comparison, computation, three dimensional space, vocabulary, tool matching, arithmetic reasoning, form matching, mark making, two pegboard tasks, and two finger dexterity board tasks. These subtests are used to define nine aptitudes: intelligence (G), verbal (V), numerical (N), spatial (S), form (P), clerical (Q), motor coordination (K), finger dexterity (F), and manual dexterity (M). Speed and accuracy are important for all the subtests. A Spanish edition is available.

Administration

The GATB may be administered individually or to a group. Some of the subtests must be given in a particular sequence. The instructions are presented orally and verbatim, preferably by one person. The manual cautions that any deviation from the written instructions may change the test and invalidate the results. Group testing should not exceed ten persons. A lower examiner-examinee ratio is recommended if examinees will require special assistance in following the instructions or if they have poor reading skills. Total time required is 2½ hours.

Special Administration Procedures for Hearing-Impaired People

The manual does not include special instructions for administration of the GATB to a hearing-impaired person. Karl, Botter, and Droege (1972) suggest the operational use of the GATB (S, P, Q, K, F, and M aptitude measures) and the Nonreading Aptitude Test Battery (NATB) for hearing-impaired persons. The Southern Test Development Field Center study (1979) indicated that the NATB should not be used as a substitute for the GATB aptitudes G, V, and N. Simple card directions were considered more fair and equitable than sign language in administering the GATB to hearing-impaired people.

Age Level

No specific ages are given. Cut-off scores are given for ninth- and tenth-grade students and for adults.

Reliability

Equivalent form and retest correlations cluster in the .80s and low .90s. Correlations are somewhat lower for the pegboard and finger dexterity subtests.

Validity

No acceptable evidence is presented to indicate that the GATB scores define levels of essential aptitudes.

Norms

The aptitude cut-offs for each occupation are derived from a fixed reference group based on test results of 4,000 persons in the 1940 U.S. working population. The group was selected according to age, sex, education, occupation, and geographic location.

Norms for Hearing-Impaired People

None have been established.

Appropriateness for Hearing-Impaired People

The GATB may be considered inappropriate for many hearing-impaired people because most subtests require verbal and reading skills, and the standardized procedures cannot be followed for all of the 12 subtests. The Southern Test Development Field Center, in an effort to standardize procedures for hearing-impaired people, has devised a card which explains each subtest. A qualified interpreter, trained to administer the GATB, is recommended.

Range of Scores

Raw scores are converted to scaled scores for each aptitude. Each job cluster has different cut-off scores for the different aptitudes. The aptitude cut-off scores for most occupations range from 85 to 115. No mean aptitude scaled score is given.

Summary of Buros Institute Publications

Discussed in the seventh edition of Buros's *Mental Measurements Yearbook* (Vol. 2, pp. 1055–1061). The GATB is the best researched of the multiple aptitude batteries, however it does not include measures of mechanical comprehension or information. The U. S. Employment Service "fails to provide empirical evidence to show superiority of the multiple cutoff approach over alternative methods" (p. 1059). No indication is given of the relative probabilities of success for the individual who qualifies for more than one occupation-aptitude profile. The aptitudes are not measured independently. In spite of its limitations, the GATB can be a useful tool for vocational counselors.

General References

Bemis, S., Bonner, R., Kearney, T., & VonLobsdorf, K. Development of a new occupational aptitude structure for the GATB. *Vocational Guidance Quarterly*, 1973, *22*(2), 130-135.

Bemis, S., Bonner, R., Kearney, T., & VonLobsdorf, K. The new occupational aptitude pattern structure for the GATB. *Vocational Guidance Quarterly*, 1973, *22*(3), 189-194.

Hull, M., & Halloran, W. The validity of the NATB for the mentally handicapped. *Education and Psychological Measurement*, 1976, *36*(2), 547-552.

U. S. Employment Service, Division of Testing Staff. Ten years of USES research on the disadvantaged. *Vocational Guidance Quarterly*, 1978, *26*(4), 334-341.

Watts, F., & Everitt, B. The factorial structure of the general aptitude test battery. *Journal of Clinical Psychology*, 1980, *36*(3), 763-767.

References Related to Hearing-Impaired People

Karl, F., Botter, R., & Droege, R. GATB aptitude testing of the deaf: Problems & possibilities. *Journal of Employment Counseling*, March 1972, 14-19.

Sanderson, R. Preparation of the hearing impaired for an adult vocational life. *Journal of Rehabilitation of the Deaf*, 1973, *6*(3), 12-18.

Southern Test Development Field Center. *The development of GATB administration procedures for the deaf*. Raleigh: U.S. Dept. of Labor, Employment and Training Administration, 1979.

GENERAL CLERICAL TEST

Author
G. K. Bennett

Publisher
The Psychological Corporation
757 Third Avenue
New York, NY 10017

Price
$53.00 (package of 100 tests)

Date of Edition
1944

General Purpose
The General Clerical Test (GCT) is designed to measure vocational aptitudes important in clerical-related occupations.

Description
The GCT consists of one booklet containing nine subtests: *checking, alphabetizing, arithmetic computation, error location, arithmetic reasoning, spelling, reading comprehension, vocabulary,* and *grammar*. These subtests may be used, singly or in combination, to appraise the suitability of an applicant for a given job or to assign an inexperienced person to appropriate work.

Administration
The GCT may be administered individually or to a group. The timing for each of the nine subtests varies; the full test requires 47 minutes.

Special Administration Procedures for Hearing-Impaired People
No special administration procedures for hearing-impaired people have been established. Repetition of the instructions is encouraged. Instructions for the GCT may be given in sign language or gesture if necessary without upsetting standardized administration procedures.

Age Level
Grades 9 through 16 and "average young adults"

Reliability

Test-retest coefficients of the nine subtests of the GCT ranged from .59 to .88. An overall reliability coefficient of .94 is reported in the manual.

Validity

The manual reports concurrent validity studies using the Wonderlic Personnel Test administered to 1,589 people. The validity coefficients ranged from .54 to .83. The GCT was also analyzed with a sample of 278 people using the Minnesota Clerical Test. Correlations in this case ranged from .36 to .67.

Norms for Hearing-Impaired People

None have been established.

Appropriateness for Hearing-Impaired People

The vocabulary subtest may be inappropriate for many hearing-impaired people. All other subtests are based on clerical and numerical abilities. The test is designed for "average young adults." Therefore, validity of overall results may be in question when administering the test to anyone not representative of this generic group. Comparison of results with hearing-impaired people in general clerical-related occupations is not possible.

Range of Scores

Raw scores are converted to percentiles.

Interpretation

The test can provide an estimate of a person's ability to handle clerical tasks (with appropriate training).

Summary of Buros Institute Publications

Reviewed in the eighth edition of Buros's *Mental Measurements Yearbook* (Vol. 2, pp. 1652-1653). The GCT compares favorably with similar tests. Norm tables are more extensive than most, but racial, ethnic, and age differences need attention. For those willing to take the time and trouble to compile local normative and validity data, this test should be considered.

General References

Doppelt, J. E., & Seashore, H. G. How effective are your tests? *Test Service Bulletin* (No. 37). New York: The Psychological Corporation, June 1949.

Hughes, J. L., & McNamara, W. J. Relationship of short employment tests and general clerical tests. *Personnel Psychology*, 1955, *8*, 331-337.

References Related to Hearing-Impaired People

None available

96 / Assessment of Hearing-Impaired People

MINNESOTA CLERICAL TEST

Author
D. M. Andrew, D. G. Paterson, and H. Longstaff

Publisher
The Psychological Corporation
757 Third Avenue
New York, NY 10017

Price
$24.00 (package of 100 tests)

Date of Edition
1959 (revised)

General Purpose
The Minnesota Clerical Test (MCT) is a test of speed and accuracy in performing clerical-related work. It has been found useful for selecting clerical employees and for advising those who seek clerical training.

Description
The MCT consists of two parts, *number checking* and *name checking*. In each part there are 200 items consisting of 100 identical and 100 dissimilar pairs. The examinee is asked to check the identical pairs. The numbers in number checking range from 3 through 12 digits, and the names in name checking contain from 7 through 17 letters. Separate time limits are used for the two parts. Exact dialogue for the administrator is provided in the manual.

Administration
The MCT may be administered individually or to a group. A stopwatch or other satisfactory device is needed to time the two parts. Total testing time is 15 minutes.

Special Administration Procedures for Hearing-Impaired People
No special administration procedures for hearing-impaired people have been established. Instructions for the test may be administered in sign language or by demonstration if necessary without upsetting standardized administration procedures.

Age Level
14 years (grade 8) and above

Reliability
The reliability coefficients provided are based on three studies using the test-retest method. In all instances, there was a considerable time interval between successive testings. The three studies utilized 28 students in commercial training courses, 48 university business students, 36 bank/bookkeeping machine operators, and 136 clerks (all women). The reliability coefficients provided from all three studies range from .56 to .93 for the number checking section and .62 to .86 for the name checking section.

Validity
Several validity coefficients are provided. A coefficient of .65 is reported based upon the relationship between test scores and personal history ratings of clerical workers. Coefficients from .55 to .71 are reported between MCT scores and scores on three clerical and two mental ability tests.

Norms
Norms are based on the performance of 25 industrial groups and two school groups. The industrial groups are classified according to sex, status (applicant or employee), geographical location, and place of employment. An extensive and careful sampling of St. Paul, Minn., public school pupils (grades 8 to 12) comprises the first school group. The second school group consists of eleventh and twelfth grade students classified according to their high school curriculum. This group is a cross-section sampling of 6,262 pupils from 76 representative New England high schools.

Norms for Hearing-Impaired People
None have been established.

Appropriateness for Hearing-Impaired People

Because percentile ranks for young adults (13 to 18 years of age) are presented by grade levels 8 through 12, interpretation of scores for hearing-impaired adolescents may be difficult due to variations in class placements. More important, hearing-impaired people are not included in any existing norm groups. Comparison of scores with hearing-impaired people in existing clerical positions is impossible. Local relevant norms would need to be developed.

Range of Scores

The raw score for each section is the number of items correct minus the number wrong. The maximum raw score is 200. Raw scores are converted to percentiles for different norm groups.

Interpretation

Test results are used primarily for decisions of vocational training and placement.

Summary of Buros Institute Publications

Discussed in the fifth edition of Buros's *Mental Measurements Yearbook* (pp. 871-874). The reviewers commend the MCT as a very acceptable and usable test for selection of promising clerical workers and for guidance in the selection of students for clerical training. However, for better prediction of clerical success, it is suggested that supplemental tests be administered to identify additional abilities (i.e., computation, spelling, alphabetizing, or vocabulary).

General References

Andrew, D. M. Analysis of the Minnesota Vocational Test for clerical workers, I and II. *Journal of Applied Psychology*, 1937, *21*, 18-47; 139-172.

Hay, E. N. Crossvalidation of clerical aptitude tests. *Journal of Applied Psychology*, 1950, *34*, 153-158.

Hay, E. N. Mental ability in clerical selection. *Journal of Applied Psychology*, 1951, *35*, 250-251.

References Related to Hearing-Impaired People

None available

MINNESOTA RATE OF MANIPULATION TESTS

Author

W. A. Zeigler

Publisher

American Guidance Service, Inc.
Publishers Building
Circle Pines, MN 55014

Price

$105.00 per test kit (two test boards, blocks, manual, carrying case, and 50 test forms)

Date of Edition

1969

General Purpose

The battery of the Minnesota Rate of Manipulation Tests (MRMT) is designed to measure manual dexterity. Its purpose is to help employers improve the efficiency of personnel selection for jobs requiring arm and hand dexterity.

Description

The MRMT consists of five subtests: the *Placing Test, Turning Test, Displacing Test, One-Hand Turning and Placing Test,* and *Two-Hand Turning and Placing Test.* The first two subtests are the most widely used. Each subtest requires the individual to place blocks into the holes of a board in some specified manner.

Administration

The MRMT may be administered individually or to a group. If the MRMT is to be used as a basis for employee selection, it must be administered identically to all applicants. The client stands at a table throughout the administration of the MRMT. The testing table should be between 28 and 32 inches in height. A watch which measures seconds is needed. Separate directions are given for administering the Turning Test and the Displacing Test to the blind. Test trials are permitted. When the MRMT is administered to a group, the examiner should demonstrate the tasks on a separate form board while reading the directions to the group. Total time required is 45 minutes.

Special Administration Procedures for Hearing-Impaired People

No special administration procedures for hearing-impaired people have been established. The test should be administered individually. Instructions can be altered to meet the communication needs of hearing-impaired people. There are special administration procedures for blind people, consisting primarily of additional practice trials.

Age Level

13 years and above

Reliability

Jurgensen (1943) determined reliability on four subtests of the MRMT (Placing, Turning, One-Hand Turning and Placing, and Two-Hand Placing and Turning) by correlating time on first and second trials and correcting with the Spearman-Brown formula. The reliability coefficients ranged from .87 to .95. With the four-trial testing, the reliability coefficients for 212 persons ranged from .93 to .98.

Validity

Jurgensen (1943) conducted research on the validity of the MRMT. Four MRMT subtests were compared with success criteria of manufacturing employees as rated by supervisors. The following correlations were obtained: Placing, .32; Turning, .46; One-Hand Turning and Placing, .57; and Two-Hand Turning and Placing, .33.

Norms

The norms are based on the distribution of scores obtained from 3,000 people tested by the Employment Stabilization Research Institute at the University of Minnesota. The sample consisted largely of unemployed, older adults of the Depression era.

Norms for Hearing-Impaired People

None have been established.

Appropriateness for Hearing-Impaired People

The MRMT test items are appropriate for hearing-impaired people. The major disadvantage of the test is that the results cannot be compared with other hearing-impaired people.

Range of Scores

Raw scores are converted to percentiles, standard scores, and stanines for each of the subtests.

Interpretation

The MRMT test results are used primarily to evaluate potential for vocational training and vocational placement. The test is often used for rehabilitation evaluation and prescriptive planning.

Summary of Buros Institute Publications

Discussed in the seventh edition of Buros's *Mental Measurements Yearbook* (Vol. 2, pp. 1482–1483). The reviewers feel that, in spite of several deficiencies, the MRMT is a valuable aid in vocational placement decisions. There are inadequate norms and validity information. The potential user would be wise to develop job-specific norms.

General References

Jurgensen, C. E. Extension of the Minnesota Rate of Manipulation Test. *Journal of Applied Psychology*, 1943, *27*, 164–169.

Paterson, D. G., Elliott, R. M., et al. *Minnesota Mechanical Ability Tests*. Minneapolis: University of Minnesota Press, 1930.

Roberts, J. R., & Bauman, M. K. *Motor skills tests adapted to the blind.* Minneapolis: Educational Test Bureau, 1944.

References Related to Hearing-Impaired People

None available

O'CONNER FINGER DEXTERITY TEST
and
O'CONNER TWEEZER DEXTERITY TEST

Author
J. O'Conner

Publisher
Stoelting Company
1350 S. Kostner Avenue
Chicago, IL 60623

Price
Finger Dexterity Test: $58.00 (set and manual)
Tweezer Dexterity Test: $58.00 (set and manual)

Date of Edition
1926 (Finger Dexterity Test)
1928 (Tweezer Dexterity Test)

General Purpose
Both the Finger Dexterity Test (FDT) and the Tweezer Dexterity Test (TDT) are designed to measure finger manipulation and eye-hand coordination. Their purpose is to determine vocational aptitude for small-parts manipulation.

Description
Each test consists of a board with rows of small holes and a well containing small metal pins. The FDT has larger holes to hold three pins each. The TDT has smaller holes for only one pin each and also has tweezers. The tweezer task requires finer coordination and thus provides finer discriminations between the examinees.

Administration
Both tests are administered individually, and the tasks are timed. The examinee sits at a table about 30 inches high with the board placed before him/her. The person may change the angle of the board if desired. Only one hand is to be used. The examiner explains the task and demonstrates it. The examinee is allowed to fill exactly 10 practice holes. After a short rest, the person fills the rest of the board with pins, using fingers for the FDT and tweezers for the TDT. For the tweezer task, the total time required to fill the board is recorded. For the finger task, the times required to fill the first 50 holes and the second 50 holes are recorded separately. Each test requires 8 to 16 minutes.

Special Administration Procedures for Hearing-Impaired People
No special administration procedures for hearing-impaired people have been established. Instructions for the test may be given through sign language, gestures, or demonstration if necessary without upsetting standardized administration procedures.

Age Level
14 years and above

Reliability
No data is provided in the manual.

Validity
No data is provided in the manual. Generalizations are made that workers in various assembly jobs have higher average scores than the general population. Therefore the tests should distinguish between those who have this aptitude and those who do not.

Norms
Normative data and population are not adequately described. Norms are presumably based on different groups of male and female factory employees and applicants. Average scores on the FDT are also given for meter and instrument assemblers (female only), bank tellers, garage mechanics, skilled workers, semiskilled workers, and butter wrappers.

Norms for Hearing-Impaired People
None have been established.

Appropriateness for Hearing-Impaired People
The tests themselves are motor tasks requiring no verbal skills. Both tests seem to be appropriate for hearing-impaired people. Results cannot be compared with other hearing-impaired workers in similar jobs.

Range of Scores

Raw scores are converted to stanines, percentiles, and letter grades. For the FDT, stanine scores range from 2.0 to 8.0. For the TDT, stanine scores range from 2.5 to 7.5.

Interpretation

Individual scores—converted to stanine, percentile, and/or letter scores—are compared to norms provided in the manual. Each examiner should decide what is a desirable level of performance for a given occupation.

Summary of Buros Institute Publications

Discussed in the 1940 edition of Buros's *Mental Measurements Yearbook* (pp. 435, 455). The reviewers expressed a need for more validity and reliability data presented in convenient and standard form. They suggest that the tests may be useful in the selection of shopworkers, watchmakers, and workers in various assembly jobs.

General References

Gluskinos, U., & Brennan, T. F. Selection and evaluation procedures for operating room personnel. *Journal of Applied Psychology*, 1971, *55*(2), 165-169.

Hayes, E. G. Selecting women for shop work. *Personnel Journal*, 1932, *11*, 69-85.

Hines, M., & O'Conner, J. A measure of finger dexterity. *Personnel Journal*, 1926, *4*, 379-382.

References Related to Hearing-Impaired People

Norden, K. The structure of abilities in a group of deaf adolescents. *Education and Psychology Interactions* (Sweden), 1970, *32*, 1-22.

PURDUE PEGBOARD

Author
J. Tiffin

Publisher
Science Research Associates
259 E. Erie Street
Chicago, IL 60611

Price
$85.80 (pegboard and manual)

Date of Edition
1968

General Purpose

The Purdue Pegboard is a test of manual and finger dexterity designed to aid in the selection of employees for industrial jobs such as packing, assembling, operation of certain machines, and other manual jobs. The test measures dexterity for two types of activity: one involving gross movements of hands, fingers, and arms; and the other involving primarily what might be called fingertip dexterity.

Description

The pegboard has a double row of holes. At the top of the board are four bins holding plugs, collars, washers, and pegs. The test consists of four parts: putting pegs from the right-hand cup into the right-hand row of holes using the right hand; a similar task for the left hand; using both hands to put pegs in simultaneously; and an assembly task consisting of inserting a peg with the right hand, a washer with the left hand, a collar with the right, and another washer with the left.

Administration

The Purdue Pegboard may be administered individually or to a group. The examinee is not required to read anything. Demonstrations are done by the examiner before each test. Each person must practice each step before the test actually begins. The total time required is 30 minutes.

Special Administration Procedures for Hearing-Impaired People

No guidelines are provided to indicate special administration procedures for hearing-impaired people. However, the instructions are demonstrated and therefore should not be a problem for most hearing-impaired people. Demonstration may be supplemented by sign language and/or pantomime.

Age Level

Grade 9 through college and adults

Reliability

Reliability data in the manual indicates that test-retest reliability correlations for the one-trial administration range from .60 to .76 with a median of .68. According to the Spearman-Brown formula, estimated reliabilities for the three-trial scores ranged from .84 to .90. Stepping up the reliability coefficient to the three-trial length raises the median to .86.

Validity

The authors state that the scores have satisfactory validity. They further state that, under certain circumstances, correlations as low as .20 may be considered as evidence of adequate validity for a test of this sort. No further information regarding validity is provided in the manual.

Norms

Separate norms are provided for male industrial applicants, military veterans, and college students. Norms for women are based on a combined group of college students and industrial applicants. No information is given concerning the composition of these groups relative to specific industry, task involvement, or age.

Norms for Hearing-Impaired People

None have been established.

Appropriateness for Hearing-Impaired People

The performance nature of the test items makes the Purdue Pegboard appropriate for hearing-impaired people. Comparison of test results with other hearing-impaired people, however, is not possible. Therefore, one must be cautious in interpreting results.

Range of Scores

Scores are included for right hand, left hand, both hands, and assembly. The number of pins inserted and the number of parts assembled is the total raw score. Raw scores are converted to percentiles.

Interpretation

In a school situation, this test can be used to measure manual dexterity of students. In a rehabilitation setting, test results can be used to assess applicants for small-parts assembly-line work.

Summary of Buros Institute Publications

Discussed in Buros's *Vocational Tests and Reviews* (pp. 557-558). The reviewers are critical of its lack of validity. The manual provides limited evidence to justify its use as a selective device for vocational guidance. They recommend that further research be conducted on the population for which the test is to be used. They also recommend revision of the manual to include more significant information.

General References

Long, L., & Hill, J. Additional norms for the Purdue Pegboard. *Occupations*, 1947, *26*, 160-161.

Siegel, M., & Hirschborn, B. Adolescent norms for the Purdue Pegboard tests. *Personnel and Guidance Journal*, 1958, 36, 363-365.

Tiffin, J., & Asher, E. J. The Purdue Pegboard: Norms and studies of reliability and validity. *Journal of Applied Psychology*, 1948, *32*, 234-237.

References Related to Hearing-Impaired People

Bolton, B. An alternative solution for the factor analysis of communication skills and nonverbal abilities of deaf clients. *Education and Psychological Measurement*, 1973, *33*(2), 459-463.

Nowell, R. F., & Stuckless, E. R. An interpreter training program. *Journal of Rehabilitation of the Deaf*, 1974, *7*(3), 69-73.

Rapin, I. The Purdue Pegboard as a screening test for brain damage and mental retardation in nonverbal children. *Volta Review*, 1967, *69*(10), 635-638.

REVISED MINNESOTA PAPER FORM BOARD TEST

Author
R. Likert and W. H. Quasha

Publisher
The Psychological Corporation
757 Third Avenue
New York, NY 10017

Price
Forms AA, BB: $7.65 per package (25 tests, manual, and scoring stencil)
Forms MA, MB: $5.50 per package (50 answer sheets); $2.00 per set of scoring stencils

Date of Edition
1970

General Purpose
The Revised Minnesota Paper Form Board Test (MPFB-R) is designed to measure those aspects of mechanical ability requiring visualization and manipulation of objects in space. Test performance appears to be related to general intelligence.

Description
The MPFB-R is a speed test of 64 two-dimensional diagrams cut into separate parts. For each diagram there are five figures with lines indicating the different shapes out of which they are made. From these, the examinee chooses the one figure which is composed of the exact parts shown in the original diagram. The MPFB-R is presented in four series: AA and BB, and MA and MB. Series MA and AA have identical content, as do series MB and BB.

Administration
The MPFB-R may be administered individually or to a group. Directions are read aloud while examinees read them visually. Test booklets, answer sheets (when using Series MA and MB), and pencils are supplied. Following the completion of four sample problems and subsequent corrections, the examinee proceeds independently for the full test. Total time required is approximately 20 minutes.

Special Administration Procedures for Hearing-Impaired People
No special administration procedures for hearing-impaired people have been established. Test instructions may be given through sign language or demonstration if necessary without upsetting standardized administration procedures.

Age Level
Grades 9 through 12 and adults

Reliability
Reliability coefficients determined by a test-retest method range from .71 to .78 with standard errors of measurement ranging from 3.1 to 4.5.

Validity
Concurrent validity measures reveal the strongest correlation of the MPFB-R with tests of spatial ability (.38 to .70). Other validity correlations were reported with tests of general intelligence (.04 to .71); numerical ability (.16 to .55); mechanical ability (.09 to .47); verbal ability (.10 to .45); and clerical ability (.17 to .51).

Norms
Percentile norms for the MPFB-R are available for a variety of educational and industrial groups. Educational group norms are based on more than 38,000 male and female high school students and engineering students. The students, from varying socioeconomic levels and races, resided in Iowa, Minnesota, Illinois, Utah, Kentucky, and New England. Industrial group norms are based on more than 900 female applicants for employment as machine operators, inspectors, and assemblers, and more than 6,800 male applicants and employees in electrical and mechanical work, drafting, engineering, science, and factory production. These people resided in Pennsylvania, New York, Michigan, Ohio, Minnesota, Delaware, Missouri, and Maryland.

Norms for Hearing-Impaired People
None have been established.

Appropriateness for Hearing-Impaired People

The tasks required in the test are nonverbal and therefore manageable by most hearing-impaired people. Comparison of results with other hearing-impaired people in mechanical occupations is not possible.

Range of Scores

Raw scores are converted to percentiles.

Interpretation

The higher the percentile ranking, the greater the person's spatial ability and potential for success in vocational areas requiring such ability.

Summary of Buros Institute Publications

Discussed in the fifth edition of Buros's *Mental Measurements Yearbook* (pp. 911-912). According to the reviewers, the test appears to be useful even if it is regarded merely as a general test of cognitive capacity in a nonverbal medium.

General References

Altender, L. E. The value of intelligence, personality and vocational interests in a guidance program. *Journal of Educational Psychology*, 1940, *31*, 449-459.

Bennett, G. C., & Cruickshank, R. M. *A summary of manual and mechanical ability tests*. New York: The Psychological Corporation, 1942.

Dicken, C. F., & Black, J. D. Predictive validity of psychometric evaluations of supervisors. *Journal of Applied Psychology*, 1965, *49*, 34-47.

References Related to Hearing-Impaired People

Bolton, B. An alternative solution for the factor analysis of communication skills and nonverbal abilities of deaf clients. *Education and Psychological Measurement*, 1973, *33*(2), 459-463.

7

VOCATIONAL INTEREST TESTS

GEIST PICTURE INTEREST INVENTORY (REVISED)

Author
H. Geist

Publisher
Western Psychological Services
12031 Wilshire Boulevard
Los Angeles, CA 90025

Price
$9.50 per kit (10 Form M and 10 Form F test booklets, manual, and motivation questionnaire)
$4.50 (manual)
$8.50 (25 Form M test booklets)
$7.50 (25 Form F test booklets)

Date of Edition
1971 (revised)

General Purpose
The Geist Picture Interest Inventory (GPII) was developed with the idea of de-emphasizing the "considerable verbal proficiency" usually required of interest inventory examinees. The GPII uses pictures (drawings) to assess the occupational and avocational interests of males and females. The test also seeks to identify motivating forces behind occupational choice.

Description
The test includes booklets of picture triads and motivation questionnaires. There are some separate booklets and questionnaires for males and females. The triads fall into 12 categories in terms of general interest areas: persuasive, clerical, mechanical, musical, scientific, outdoor, literary, computational, artistic, social service, dramatic, and personal service (female only).

Administration

The GPII is designed to be administered individually. The Form M booklet contains 44 triads of drawings for males; Form F contains 27 triads of drawings for females. These drawings picture major vocations and avocations. The examinee is asked to circle the preferred occupation among those shown. When finished, the examinee is asked to indicate the reasons for circling each picture. The reasons for making choices fall under seven motivational areas: could not say, family, prestige, financial, intrinsic and personality, environmental, past experience. Total time required ranges from 30 to 45 minutes.

Special Administration Procedures for Hearing-Impaired People

There is a special edition of the GPII for hearing-impaired males, the Geist Picture Interest Inventory: Deaf: Male Form (GPII:D:M). Directions for taking the GPII:D:M are simplified to the fourth grade reading level, and there are no questions under each triad of pictures. The GPII:D:M is also self-administering for most people, but directions may be presented in sign language or any other possible mode of communication if necessary.

Age Level

Grades 8 to 16

Reliability

Test-retest coefficients of reliability for the 11 male GPII interests exist for 15 different groups. These correlations are said to be "at high levels of statistical significance;" the median correlation coefficients for the 11 interests range from .58 to .87. A smaller group of females (six groups) provided test-retest correlation coefficients with medians ranging from .67 to .81.

Validity

In an effort to show validity, the test author compared 10 of 11 GPII interests to the 10 interests on the Kuder Occupational Interest Survey. Leaving out the remedial reading groups, the validity coefficients ranged from .24 to .66. There were several negative correlations in remedial reading groups which the author interpreted to his advantage, stating that examinees with reading problems respond more validly to the GPII than to verbal interest inventories.

Research data are also available on correlation with grades, comparison of parent ratings with scores on interest scales, and a five-year follow-up study on the the initial standardization group in terms of work satisfaction. Some interest scales have been shown to be predictive of success in certain subjects. Almost all GPII interest scales correlated highly with parents' ratings of their children's interests. Twenty percent of the initial standardization group were followed up five years later. Using various criteria—entrance into an occupation and length of time in that occupation, college major, and satisfaction or dissatisfaction with current work—all GPII interest scales were found to be valid.

Norms

The population tested for the GPII included 1,289 males and 465 females representing remedial reading groups, trade schools, high schools, and colleges (rural, urban, and suburban). Students at Puerto Rican and Hawaiian high schools and colleges were included. There are also occupational norms for both males and females in a variety of occupational groups.

Norms for Hearing-Impaired People

The population samples for GPII:D:M were drawn from 20 residential schools for the deaf, vocational rehabilitation centers in 26 states, seven public schools, Gallaudet College, and a group of employed deaf males (number not specified) as follows:

Residential Schools	1,029
Vocational Rehabilitation Services	897
Public Day Schools	122
Gallaudet College	123
Total	2,171

Appropriateness for Hearing-Impaired People

The GPII:D:M appears to be appropriate for hearing-impaired males because of the performance nature of the test. However, the norms for hearing-impaired people are dated. Public day school males and employed males are under-represented in the existing norm sample.

Range of Scores

The test is scored by counting the number of times each of the 12 occupational interest areas are selected. Raw scores are converted to *T*-scores for males/females according to age, education, location, and membership in special groups.

Interpretation

A *T*-score above 70 usually indicates that a person has a high interest in that particular occupational area. A *T*-score under 30 indicates that he/she does not like or enjoy activites in that occupational area. Graphs are provided which profile 11 male and female occupational groups. These results can be used by vocational counselors to assist people in determining occupational or career choices and the motivation behind such choices. The actual test drawings can be used to elicit client stories which can help counselors gain insight into attitudes toward work, family relationships, and occupational rejection.

A *T*-score above 60 in any of the seven motivation areas is considered a significant indicator of strong occupational motivation. Very high or very low motivation scores should be examined closely

Summary of Buros Institute Publications

Reviewed in the sixth edition of Buros's *Mental Measurements Yearbook* (pp. 1272–1277). The reviewers are in agreement in cautioning against use of the GPII in direct guidance situations. It may have possibilities as a clinical tool with poor readers. Further research is recommended.

General References

Geist, H. Work satisfaction and scores on a picture interest inventory. *Journal of Applied Psychology*, 1963, *47*, 369–373.

Montesano, N., & Geist, H. Differences in reasons for occupational choices between 9th and 12th grade boys. *Personnel and Guidance Journal*, 1964, *43*, 127–134.

Tiedeman, D.U. Testing the test: Geist Picture Interest Inventory. *Personnel and Guidance Journal*, 1960, *38*, 506–507.

References Related to Hearing-Impaired People

Bolton, B. A critical review of the Geist Picture Interest Inventory: Deaf Form: Male. *Journal of Rehabilitation of the Deaf*, 1971 *5*(2), 21–29.

Geist, H. Occupational interest profiles of the deaf. *Personnel and Guidance Journal*, 1962, *41*, 50–55.

Geist, H. *The Geist Picture Interest Inventory: Deaf Form: Male*. Los Angeles: Western Psychological Services, 1962.

Picture Interest Exploration Survey

Author
F. Mahoney

Publisher
Education Achievement Corporation
P.O. Box 7310
Waco, TX 76710

Price
$350.00 (see description)

Date of Edition
1974

General Purpose
The Picture Interest Exploration Survey (PIES) is a career-interest inventory presented in a visual, nonreading format. It is designed to help students investigate their vocational interests and apply this information to their career goals.

Description
Components of the PIES include 160 color slides, two slide trays, one audio tape, two sets of career reference cards, one student-teacher manual, and 50 student response sheets. The uniqueness of the PIES is that all slides are of people's *hands* performing the occupational tasks. This is done to diminish cultural and sexual biases.

Administration
The PIES is designed to be administered in a classroom setting. Each student is given a response sheet. As the numbered slides are presented, the student circles the corresponding number on the response sheet to indicate those occupational tasks that he or she finds interesting. At the conclusion of the slide presentation, the student counts the number of circles he or she has drawn in each of the 13 rows. Total time required is one hour.

Special Administration Procedures for Hearing-Impaired People
No special administration procedures for hearing-impaired people have been established. There are no reading requirements, and students need not be familiar with terminology of the world of work in order to respond accurately to test items.

Age Level
Seventh grade to adulthood

Reliability
The PIES is a relatively new survey and needs to be evaluated for reliability.

Validity
Validation information is available from Education Achievement Corporation for a nominal fee.

Norms
No norms are provided because, by design, PIES does not compare examinees' scores.

Norms for Hearing-Impaired People
None have been established.

Appropriateness for Hearing-Impaired People
The PIES appears to be appropriate for hearing-impaired people. It is presented visually, does not require high reading skills, gives immediate feedback, and is easy to administer and score. Norms for hearing-impaired people are not relevant because of the design of the test.

Range of Scores
A person's scores for each of the 13 rows are compared with his or her overall average score. A score on any of the 13 rows which is two or more points above the person's average score is considered high; a score two or more points below the average is considered low. An individual's average score is computed by dividing the total score by 13.

Interpretation

Rows with high scores indicate the career clusters in which the student is most interested and perhaps most knowledgeable. Rows with low scores indicate career clusters in which the student has little or no interest or knowledge.

Summary of Buros Institute Publications

The PIES has not been reviewed in Buros's *Mental Measurements Yearbooks*.

General References

Careers research monographs. Chicago: The Institute for Research, 1972.

Valuing approach to career education (The 6-8 Series). Waco, Tex.: Education Achievement Corporation, 1973.

Vital information for education and work (VIEW). Bloomington, Ind.: National Center for Career Information Services, 1968.

References Related to Hearing-Impaired People

None available

STRONG-CAMPBELL INTEREST INVENTORY

Author
E. K. Strong and D. P. Campbell

Publisher
Stanford University Press
Stanford, CA 94305

Price
$10.50 (manual)
$8.70 (specimen set of inventory booklets)

Date of Edition
1981 (revised scoring, Form T325)

General Purpose

The Strong-Campbell Interest Inventory (SCII) is a revised edition of the Strong Vocational Interest Blank. The revision merges the male and female forms and provides a theoretical framework (Holland's Theory) for layout of the interest profile and interpretation of the scores. The SCII's principal function is to provide information about people and their relationship to the working world which will aid them in making decisions about the course of their lives.

Description

The test consists of an inventory booklet listing 325 items to which the person responds with "like," "indifferent," or "dislike." Scoring scales consist of six general occupational themes, 23 basic interest scales, and 162 occupational scales. Scores help to identify patterns of a person's interests and to show the degree of similarity between a person's interests and those of workers in a wide range of occupations.

Administration

The SCII may be administered individually or to a group. Instructions are written on the test booklet. The person is instructed to work quickly and to answer every item. A pre-test orientation is suggested to explain the purpose of the test. Total testing time ranges from 30 to 40 minutes.

Special Administration Procedures for Hearing-Impaired People

No special administration procedures for hearing-impaired people have been established.

Age Level

The test can be used with persons from age 13 through adulthood. Because interests begin to solidify for most people at age 17 or 18, the results are more appropriate for career planning at this age level. The SCII booklet reads at about the sixth-grade level.

Reliability

Test-retest reliability correlations indicate substantial short-term stability. Variation occurs with respect to the age of the person when first tested and the length of the retest interval. For two-week, thirty-day, and three-year periods, the median test-retest correlations are .91, .89, and .87 respectively for the Occupational Scales. Test-retest correlates over similar periods for the General Occupational Themes, Basic Interest Scales, and Special Scales range from .81 to .91.

Validity

Concurrent validity, checked by comparing scores of people in different occupations, shows that the scales do separate occupations according to the Basic Interest Scales, with highest- and lowest-scoring samples about 2.5 standard deviations apart. Data include scores for more than 300 occupational samples with a median sample size of 250. Predictive validity shows considerable agreement between the scores earned and the person's eventual occupation. Some scales are less predictive than others. Consistency between scores on Basic Interest and Occupational Scales yields a greater predictive accuracy. Highest validity was found in scales where occupations are distinct and tightly defined.

Norms

Occupational samples, used as criterion groups for the development of the scales, were drawn from a wide variety of occupations with an average sample size of 248 people. The overall mean age is 39.2 years, the average level of education is 16.6 years, and the average length of experience is 12.2 years.

Norms for Hearing-Impaired People

None have been established.

Appropriateness for Hearing-Impaired People

Due to the fact the the SCII relies totally on the ability to comprehend written English at a sixth-grade reading level or above, this inventory does not appear to be appropriate for the general hearing-impaired population. Also, individual results cannot be compared to hearing-impaired people in a variety of occupations.

Range of Scores

The range, mean, and standard deviation differ for each scale of the inventory. Criterion samples have been converted to a T-score distribution with a mean of 50 and standard deviation of 10.

Interpretation

Counselor and client may review a computer-printed profile to determine a client's occupational interests and how an individual's interests compare with workers in a variety of occupations. This information may be used to help a person focus on special areas of interest and to make better-informed educational and career decisions.

Summary of Buros Institute Publications

Previous editions of the SCII are discussed in the eighth edition of Buros's *Mental Measurements Yearbook* (Vol. 2, pp. 1614–1631). The reviews are generally positive, citing SCII as the best inventory available. Some criticism is made of inconsistency between Basic Interest and Occupational Scales, absence of mean and standard deviation data for occupational criterion groups, and secrecy about the item content of scales for test takers.

General References

Borgen, F. H., & Harper, G. T. Predictive validity of measured vocational interests with black and white college men. *Measurement and Evaluation in Guidance*, 1973, *6*, 19-27.

Campbell, D. P., & Holland, J. L. A merger in vocational interest research: Applying Holland's theory to Strong's data. *Journal of Vocational Behavior*, 1972, *2*(4), 353-376.

Lee, D. L., & Hedahl, B. Holland's personality types applied to the SVIB Basic Interest Scales. *Journal of Vocational Behavior*, 1973, *3*, 61-68.

References Related to Hearing-Impaired People

None available

WIDE RANGE INTEREST AND OPINION TEST—REVISED

Author
J. R. Jastak and S. Jastak

Publisher
Jastak Associates, Inc.
1526 Gilpin Avenue
Wilmington, DE 19806

Price
$23.90 (manual)
$11.90 (picture book)
$9.75 (50 answer sheets)
$37.95 (set of answer keys)

Date of Edition
1979

General Purpose
The Wide Range Interest and Opinion Test—Revised (WRIOT-R) is an updated version of the 1972 WRIOT. The WRIOT-R is designed to measure work interests and attitudes of an individual for career planning.

Description
The WRIOT-R consists of sets of pictures showing people engaged in various occupational/recreational activities. There are 150 sets of three pictures. In each set the client identifies one picture of an activity he/she would most like to do, and one picture of an activity he/she would least like to do. There are 18 areas of interest: art, literature, music, drama, sales, management, office work, personal service, protective service, social service, social science, biological science, physical science, numbers, mechanics, machine operation, outdoor, and athletics.

Administration

The WRIOT-R may be administered individually or to a group. In group administration, the pictures can be presented by film/slides, and it is advisable that proctors be present to check initial responses and to make sure page (picture sets) and block numbers agree on the answer sheets. Average time for completion is 40 minutes for individual administration, and 50 to 60 minutes for group administration. For administration to visually-impaired individuals, the examiner may explain a picture using the description in the manual. No reading skills are required to complete the test.

Special Administration Procedures for Hearing-Impaired People

No special administration procedures for hearing-impaired people have been established. Procedures for administration of this test to hearing-impaired people are presently being developed (Farrugia, 1981).

Age Level

5 years through adulthood

Reliability

Reliability was determined for males and females for each of the 18 clusters of interests. Split-half reliabilities (Cureton Formula) of the 36 coefficients ranged from .82 to .95.

Validity

Validity correlations obtained between the WRIOT-R and the Geist Picture Interest Inventories for 18 interest categories resulted in coefficients ranging from −.03 to .61 ($N=100$).

Norms

Norms for the revised edition of the WRIOT are based on a sample of 9,184 people representing seven age-groups (5 to 7 years, 8 to 11, 12 to 15, 16 to 19, 20 to 24, 25 to 34, and 35 and up). There was no attempt to obtain a representative sampling; the authors considered such sampling nonessential for proper standardization. According to the authors, the sample chosen was in no way restricted to any economic, intellectual, or racial populations.

Norms for Hearing-Impaired People

None have been established.

Appropriateness for Hearing-Impaired People

The WRIOT-R, a picture inventory, was developed to avoid reliance on reading skills or verbal language understanding. It can be administered nonverbally, given appropriate skills of the evaluator. The major weakness of using the test with hearing-impaired people is in the interpretation of results. Because handicapped people, specifically hearing-impaired people, are not represented in the norm group, one cannot compare results with other handicapped people who are well-established in occupations. Representation within the norming group is of vital importance to a test of this nature.

Range of Scores

Raw scores are converted to T-scores which, for each of 14 age/sex categories, range from 21 (the negative response limit) to 80 (the positive response). This range of negative and positive interest scores was obtained by assigning numerical values to T-scores symmetrically above and below the midrange of 44 to 56. The author gives mean and standard deviation numbers for males and females in each cluster. The author also provides percentiles, standard scores, stanines, and scaled score equivalents for the T-scores.

Interpretation

The major use of the results of the WRIOT-R is in preparation for educational or vocational placement. The WRIOT-R is a useful tool for rehabilitation and guidance counselors in assisting clients with career planning.

Summary of Buros Institute Publications

The WRIOT-R has not been reviewed in Buros's *Mental Measurements Yearbooks*. The 1972 edition of the WRIOT was reviewed in the eighth edition of Buros's *Mental Measurements Yearbook* (Vol. 2, pp. 1641–1643). The reviewer feels that the WRIOT offers little new information independent of that offered in other interest surveys.

General References

Ghiselli, E. E. The validity of commonly employed occupational tests. *University of California Publication in Psychology*, 1946, *5*, 253–288.

Guilford, J. P. *Psychometric methods*. New York: McGraw-Hill, 1954.

Lunneborg, P. W., & Gerry, M. H. Sex differences in changing sex-stereotyped vocational interests. *Journal of Counseling Psychology*, 1977, *24*(3), 247–250.

References Related to Hearing-Impaired People

Farrugia, D. *A study of deaf high school students' vocational interests and attitudes*. Unpublished doctoral dissertation, Northern Illinois University, 1981.

8

WORK EVALUATION SYSTEMS

JEWISH EMPLOYMENT AND VOCATIONAL SERVICE

Author
Jewish Employment and Vocational Service

Publisher
Vocational Research Institute
1700 Sansom Street
Philadelphia, PA 19103

Price
$7,975.00 (includes Work Sample Package, training for one evaluator, and one onsite consultation)

Date of Edition
1976 (updated periodically)

General Purpose
The Jewish Employment and Vocational Service (JEVS) work samples assess aptitudes, vocational interests, and work-related behaviors of rehabilitation, minority, and school populations.

Description
The present JEVS contains 28 work samples arranged in 10 worker-trait groups which are directly related to worker-trait arrangements in the *Dictionary of Occupational Titles* (1977): handling; sorting; tending; manipulating; routine checking and recording; classifying; inspecting and stock checking; craftsmanship and related work; costuming, tailoring, and dressmaking; and drafting and related work.

Administration
The JEVS is designed to be administered individually, although a number of clients can be working on different work samples simultaneously. Work samples are administered progressively starting with the simplest samples. Instructions are provided verbally and through demonstration. Written instructions are used only when required on the jobsite. One to two weeks are required to complete the

entire system. A realistic work setting and atmosphere is stressed in the manual. Two weeks of training are required for the evaluator; this training is available from JEVS as part of the instructional package.

Special Administration Procedures for Hearing-Impaired People

No special administration procedures for hearing-impaired people have been established. The administration of many of the work samples does not necessitate verbal language and, therefore, may be used with hearing-impaired people.

Age Level

High school through adults

Reliability

No published data available

Validity

Results of validity studies conducted by the Department of Labor have not been released to the public. Research done by Nadolsky (1973) concludes that JEVS is valid for evaluation of immediate employment potential.

Norms

The original norm group (1969) consisted predominantly of young, Black males with no work history. Norms were updated in 1975 based on 880 individuals from 32 facilities (vocational rehabilitation facilities, prisons, Manpower, Goodwill Industries, and secondary schools for mentally-retarded individuals) in 15 states representing all regions of the country.

Norms for Hearing-Impaired People

No norms for hearing-impaired people have been established. However, the publisher is willing to develop norms for specific populations if raw data are provided.

Appropriateness for Hearing-Impaired People

Because JEVS work samples do not rely heavily on speech or reading skills, many of the work samples are suitable for hearing-impaired people. Use of existing normative data would appear appropriate for most samples.

Range of Scores

Time and quality of performance are given equal emphasis in scoring. The client uses a time clock for each work sample. The number of minutes needed to complete the task is transferred to a three-point scale. Carefully defined scoring criteria are provided in the manual.

Interpretation

The system uses an extensive observation summary on standardized forms which list 25 specified work-factors to observe. The evaluator notes how the individual approaches the tasks. Observations are included in a written report along with specific vocational recommendations. The evaluation report may be used in career planning or job placement.

Summary of Buros Institute Publications

The JEVS is described only briefly in the eighth edition of Buros's *Mental Measurements Yearbook* (Vol. 2, pp. 1190-1193).

General References

Dictionary of occupational titles (4th ed.). Washington, D. C.: U. S. Department of Labor, 1977.

Hurwitz, S. K., & Dibrancesca, S. Behavioral modification of the emotionally retarded deaf. *Rehabilitation Literature*, 1968, *29*(9), 258-264.

Nadolsky, J. *Vocational evaluation of the culturally disadvantaged: A comparative investigation of JEVS (Jewish Employment Vocational Service) system and a model-based system* (Final Report). Auburn, Ala.: Auburn University, 1973.

References Related to Hearing-Impaired People

None available

SINGER VOCATIONAL EVALUATION SYSTEM

Author

Singer Education Division/Career Systems

Publisher

Singer, Inc.
Education and Training Division
3750 Monroe Avenue
Rochester, NY 14603

Price

$39,945.00 (complete evaluation system)

Date of Edition

1971 (updated periodically)

General Purpose

The Singer Vocational Evaluation System (SVES) is a sampling of work simulations that approximate a broad range of selected employment fields. The present work samples relate to the "Occupational Group Arrangements" and "Worker Trait Group Arrangements" sections of the U.S. Department of Labor's *Dictionary of Occupational Titles* (1977). The primary purpose of the SVES is to test vocational aptitude. The test is used for occupational evaluation, exploration, and subsequent vocational placement.

Description

At present SVES consists of the following 25 work samples: sample making; bench assembly; drafting; electrical wiring; plumbing and pipefitting; woodworking; air conditioning and refrigeration; soldering and welding; sales processing; needle trades; masonry; sheet metal; cooking and baking; small engine service; medical services; cosmetology; data calculation; soil testing; photo lab technician; production machine operating; household and industrial wiring; filing, shipping, and receiving; packaging and materials handling; electronics assembly; and welding and brazing. Each work sample is presented in a work station—a self-contained unit with the tools, supplies, and instructions necessary to complete each task.

Administration

The SVES is designed to be administered individually, although a number of clients can be working on different work samples simultaneously. Each work sample is independent. The evaluator and participant select which appropriate programs to complete. Both the evaluator and participant are actively involved in the process. Using a filmstrip or tape, the participant follows step-by-step instructions for the tasks to be completed. As the participant completes the required tasks, the evaluator reviews the progress at various checkpoints. On completion of the sample, the participant rates his/her level of interest and performance. The evaluator rates the performance and specific characteristics related to the tasks of the job as described by the *Dictionary of Occupational Titles*. Special procedures are provided for illiterate participants, and repetition of the work activity is allowed. The average time for each work station is 2 to 2½ hours. Up to three weeks may be required to complete the evaluation.

Special Administration Procedures for Hearing-Impaired People

An adaptation of the instructional format for hearing-impaired people was developed in 1979. This adaptation consists of a visually reinforced method of instruction. To date, seven work samples have been adapted for administration to hearing-impaired people: sample making, bench assembly, small engine service, production machine operating, household and industrial wiring, packaging and materials handling, and electronics assembly. The 18 other work samples are being adapted for hearing-impaired individuals under the direction of Robert Thompson, Florida School for the Deaf, St. Augustine, Florida.

Age Level

No specific ages given

Reliability

A test-retest reliability study was conducted by Cohen and Drugo (1976). They sought to estimate reliability of the scores using a random sample of 30 educable, mentally retarded, high school students. Participants were tested twice in a four-month interval to analyze the stability of aptitude-error, aptitude-time, and interest scores over time. The aptitude-error and aptitude-time scores improved significantly over time from pre- to post-test. The interest scores showed no significant changes. A coefficient of .71 was obtained on the aptitude-error variable; a coefficient of .61 was reported for aptitude-time and composite interest variables. Consistent stability coefficients within groups on both measures indicate a moderate degree of test-retest reliability.

Validity

Gannaway and Sink (1978) demonstrated relatively strong predictive validity of the SVES in two studies. A comparison of performances on given work samples with employment in specifically related jobs provided correlation coefficients of .39 to 1.00 and .42 to .80. The coefficients obtained for work samples and employment in generally related jobs were .12 to .63 and .54 to 1.00 for the two studies. Research also indicates high face and content validity for the SVES.

Norms

Norms are based on two separate experimental groups of handicapped people: Office of Vocational Rehabilitation referrals and disadvantaged CETA referrals. The sample population is described in terms of mean age, race, and highest mean grade completed. In an updated SVES evaluator's manual (1979) new normative data is presented for all revised job samples; the manual also contains performance norms for competitively employed workers for seven job samples. Method-time-measurement standards have been compiled, and industrial norms are provided. Additional data is being researched.

Norms for Hearing-Impaired People

Norms for hearing-impaired people are being developed at the Florida School for the Deaf, St. Augustine, Florida.

Appropriateness for Hearing-Impaired People

The SVES has special value for hearing-impaired people. The system realistically simulates actual jobs and provides more than a single work-trait orientation. The applicability to job experience and work situation provides a meaningful experience for the participant. In addition, the visual instruction procedures, designed specifically for hearing-impaired clients, make this vocational evaluation system highly appropriate for many hearing-impaired clients.

Range of Scores

Time and quality norms are rated on a five-point scale. Emphasis is on the quality of the finished product.

Interpretation

Through the use of interest measures, scoring procedures, and observation of clients, occupational information and vocational recommendations can be provided to the client.

Summary of Buros Institute Publications

The SVES has not been reviewed in Buros's *Mental Measurements Yearbooks*.

General References

Botterbusch, K. F. *Comparison of seven vocational evaluation systems*. Stout, Wis.: University of Wisconsin (Stout Vocational Rehabilitation Institute, Materials Development Center), 1976.

Cohen, C., & Drugo, J. Test-retest reliability of the Singer Vocational Evaluation System. *Vocational Guidance Quarterly*, 1976, *24*(3), 267–270.

Dictionary of occupational titles (4th ed.). Washington, D. C.: U. S. Department of Labor, 1977.

Gannaway, T., & Sink, J. The relationship between the vocational evaluation system by Singer and employment success in occupational groups. *Vocational Evaluation and Work Adjustment Bulletin*, 1978, *11*(2), 38–45.

References Related to Hearing-Impaired People

Watson, D. (Ed.). *Deaf evaluation and adjustment feasibility*. New York: New York University (Deafness Research and Training Center), 1976.

Testing, Orientation and Work Evaluation in Rehabilitation

Author

The Institute for Crippled and Disabled (ICD) Rehabilitation and Research Center

Publisher

ICD Rehabilitation and Research Center
340 E. 24th Street
New York, NY 10010

Price

$325.00 (full set of written evaluation materials available to evaluators who complete two-week training session)
$180.00 (evaluator's manual)
$400.00 (two-week training course)
$8,000.00 to $10,000.00 (approximate cost to set up entire system)

Date of Edition

1959 (updated periodically)

General Purpose

The major purpose of Testing, Orientation and Work Evaluation in Rehabilitation (TOWER) is vocational evaluation and assessment of handicapped individuals.

Description

The TOWER consists of 94 work samples set up to replicate or closely simulate actual jobs. These work samples evaluate job skills in 14 major occupational areas: clerical, drafting, drawing, electronics assembly, jewelry manufacturing, leather goods, lettering, machine shop, mail clerk, optical mechanics, pantograph engraving, sewing machine operator, welding, and working assembly.

Administration

The TOWER is designed to be administered individually, although a number of clients can be working on different work samples simultaneously. The client is given samples of real work situations and is asked to do tasks required in those jobs. The instructions are written. If in the real job the instructions would be written on a seventh-grade level, then the instructions for the work sample are written at that level. The instructions give some information about the jobs that use the skills being sampled. Usually, only those work samples relating to the client's interests or job-related proficiencies are given. Up to three weeks may be required to complete the evaluation.

Special Administration Procedures for Hearing-Impaired People

No special administration procedures for hearing-impaired people have been established. Demonstration of directions and repetition of work samples, which would aid many hearing-impaired people, are permitted.

Age Level

Generally, 16 years and above

Reliability

No information presently available

Validity

The evaluator's manual reports no information on validity. Sligar (1976) reports good face validity.

Norms

The TOWER was normed on clients from the Institute for the Crippled and Disabled in New York City. Sample size and characteristics are not identified. Industrial norms are not provided.

Norms for Hearing-Impaired People

None have been developed.

Appropriateness for Hearing-Impaired People

The TOWER system can be used effectively with many hearing-impaired people when appropriate modifications of the system are made. The lack of norm data on hearing-impaired workers may be a disadvantage.

Range of Scores

Clients are rated on a number scale of one (minimal ability) to five (superior ability) for each work sample.

Interpretation

Standardized norms are used to record attendance and punctuality as well as a summary of time required and quality of results. The final report is written using a standardized narrative outline. The report is used to assist rehabilitation counselors in vocational planning for their clients.

Summary of Buros Institute Publications

The TOWER has not been reviewed in Buros's *Mental Measurements Yearbooks*.

General References

Botterbusch, K. F. *The TOWER system: A comparison of commercial vocational evaluation systems*. Stout, Wis.: University of Wisconsin (Stout Vocational Rehabilitation Institute, Materials Development Center), 1980.

Pruitt, W. A. *Vocational (work) evaluation in rehabilitation*. Menomonie, Wis.: Walter Pruitt Associates, 1977.

Rosenburg, B. TOWER: Vocational testing of the handicapped. *International Rehabilitation Review*, 1972, *13*, 14–16.

Sarkees, M. D. An overview of selected evaluation systems for use in assessing the vocational aptitudes of handicapped individuals. *Diagnostique*, 1979, *4*(1), 42–51.

TOWER: Testing, Orientation and Work Evaluation in Rehabilitation. New York: Institute for Crippled and Disabled (ICD) Rehabilitation and Research Center, 1974.

References Related to Hearing-Impaired People

Pimentel, A. T. The TOWER system as a vocational test for the deaf client. *Journal of Rehabilitation of the Deaf*, 1967, *1*, 26–31.

Sligar, S. The use of commercial work samples with a hearing-impaired population. In D. Watson (Ed.), *Deaf evaluation and adjustment feasibility*. New York: New York University (Deafness Research and Training Center), 1976.

VALPAR COMPONENT WORK SAMPLE SERIES

Author

Valpar Corporation

Publisher

Valpar Corporation
3801 E. 34th Street, Suite 105
Tucson, AZ 85713

Price

$13,565.00 for 16 work samples and manuals
$1,125.00 for complete set of 15 videotapes for hearing-impaired people
(Work samples and videotapes may be purchased separately)

Date of Edition

1974 (updated periodically)

General Purpose

The Valpar Component Work Sample Series (VCWSS) is designed for use in vocational evaluation. It provides standardized work samples which measure universal worker characteristics. The present VCWSS is keyed to the worker-traits arrangement data in the *Dictionary of Occupational Titles* (1977).

Description

The VCWSS consists of 16 work sample components: small tools (mechanical), size discrimination, numerical sorting, upper extremity range of motion, clerical comprehension and aptitude, independent problem solving, multi-level sorting, simulated assembly, whole body range of motion, tri-level measurement, eye-hand-foot coordination, soldering and inspection (electronic), money handling, integrated peer performance, electrical circuiting and print reading, and drafting.

Administration

The VCWSS is designed to be administered individually, although a number of clients can be working on different work samples simultaneously. Instructions contained in manuals for each component are presented verbally to the client. A practice period is allowed prior to administration of each work sample. No specific sequence is prescribed, nor is it necessary to administer the entire system to a client. Up to three weeks may be required to complete the evaluation.

Special Administration Procedures for Hearing-Impaired People

Instructions for administration to hearing-impaired people are available on videocassette tapes for all work sample components except integrated peer performance. These tapes were produced in cooperation with New York University, Gallaudet College, and the National Theater of the Deaf.

Age Level

None specified by the publisher; norms available for ages 16 to 60

Reliability

Test-retest reliability coefficients for the work sample components range from .80 to .97.

Validity

Research is being undertaken; validity information will be published in the *Valpar Quarterly Newsletter* as it becomes available.

Norms

Time, error, and performance norms have been derived from various occupational, educational, and disability groups for people ages 16 to 60. The groups included institutionally retarded people in sheltered, independent, or community living; Seminole Community College (Arizona); San Diego employed workers; Air Force; and Skill Center unemployed, low-income populations in the Tucson area. The VCWSS also provided methods-time measurement (MTM) norms which one can use to compare the client's performance with a computer-derived projection of how long it would take a physically and mentally "normal" person to perform the given task.

Norms for Hearing-Impaired People

Work samples 1 through 12 were recently normed on students at the residential Western Pennsylvania School for the Deaf. The norm group for each work-sample component consisted of 50 males and females, ages 16 to 20, with severe (60–75 db) to profound (75+ db) congenital hearing losses.

Appropriateness for Hearing-Impaired People

With the availability of hearing-impaired norms and videotaped standardized instructions, the majority of the VCWSS work samples are appropriate for and useful in assessing general physical abilities and vocational skills of hearing-impaired people. The availability of hearing-impaired norms for most work samples adds credibility to the VCWSS for hearing-impaired people.

Range of Scores

Time and error raw scores are converted to performance percentiles. In addition, the evaluator obtains behavioral information from observing client performance of the tasks and rating worker characteristics.

Interpretation

The results of the VCWSS are usually presented as a written report and used in conjunction with other data to make decisions regarding vocational placement and/or vocational training.

Summary of Buros Institute Publications

The VCWSS has not been reviewed in Buros's *Mental Measurements Yearbooks*.

General References

Botterbusch, K. F. *A comparison of seven vocational evaluation systems.* Stout, Wis.: University of Wisconsin (Stout Vocational Rehabilitation Institute, Materials Development Center), 1976.

Brandon, T. L., Button, W. L., Rastatter, C. J., & Ross, D. R. Valpar Component Work Sample system. In A. Sax (Ed.), Innovations in vocational evaluation and work adjustment. *Vocational Evaluation and Work Adjustment Bulletin*, 1975, 8(2), 59–63.

Dictionary of occupational titles (4th ed.). Washington, D.C.: U.S. Department of Labor, 1977.

References Related to Hearing-Impaired People

Sligar, S. The use of commercial work samples with a hearing-impaired population. In D. Watson (Ed.), *Deaf evaluation and adjustment feasibility*. New York: New York University (Deafness Research and Training Center), 1976.

APPENDIX A

SUPPLEMENTARY READING ON GENERAL ASPECTS OF EVALUATING HEARING-IMPAIRED PEOPLE

Altshuler, K. Z. The social and psychological development of the deaf child: Problems, their treatment and prevention. *American Annals of the Deaf*, 1974, *119*(4), 365-376.

Altshuler, L. Psychological considerations in the school age deaf. *American Annals of the Deaf*, 1962, *107*(5), 553-559.

Arkell, C. Assessment of multiply handicapped deaf students for program development. *American Annals of the Deaf*, 1981, *126*(5), 526-532.

Barrett, S. S. Assessment of vision in the programs for the deaf. *American Annals of the Deaf*, 1979, *124*(6), 745-752.

Berlinsky, S. Measurement of the intelligence and personality of the deaf: A review of the literature. *Journal of Speech and Hearing Disorders*, 1952, *17*(2), 39-54.

Bolton, B. (Ed.). *Psychology of deafness for rehabilitation counselors*. Baltimore: University Park Press, 1976.

Bradway, K. P. Social competence of exceptional children: The deaf, the blind, and the crippled. *Exceptional Children*, 1937, *4*, 64-69.

Brenner, L., & Thompson, R. The use of projective techniques in personality evaluation of deaf adults. *Journal of Rehabilitation of the Deaf*, 1967, *1*(2), 17-30.

Burchard, E., & Myklebust, H. R. A comparison of congenital and adventitious deafness with respect to its effect on intelligence, personality and social maturity. *American Annals of the Deaf*, 1942, *87*(2), 140-154.

Cantor, D. W., & Spragins, A. Delivery of psychological services to the hearing-impaired child in the elementary school. *American Annals of the Deaf*, 1977, *122*(3), 330-336.

Craig, W. N., & Barkuloo, H. W. *Psychologists to deaf children: A developing perspective*. Pittsburgh: University of Pittsburgh Press, 1968.

Cutler, E. M. Summary of psychological experiments with the deaf. *American Annals of the Deaf*, 1941, *86*(2), 181-193.

Donoghue, R. J. The deaf personality: A study in contrasts. *Journal of Rehabilitation of the Deaf,* 1968, *2*(3), 37-51.

Donoghue, R. J., & Bolton, B. Psychological evaluation of deaf rehabilitation clients. *Journal of Rehabilitation of the Deaf,* 1971, *5*(1), 29-38.

Furth, H. G. Research with the deaf: Implications for language and cognition. *Psychological Bulletin, 1964, 62*(3), 145-163.

Garrett, J. F., & Levine, E. S. *Psychological practices with the physically disabled.* New York: Columbia University Press, 1969.

Grinker, R. R. (Ed.). *Psychiatric diagnosis, therapy, and research on the psychotic deaf.* Washington, D.C.: U.S. Department of Health, Education, and Welfare (Social and Rehabilitation Service), 1971.

Hess, D. W. Evaluation of the young deaf adult. *Journal of Rehabilitation of the Deaf,* 1969, *3*(2), 6-21.

Hood, H. B. A preliminary survey of some mental abilities of deaf children. *British Journal of Educational Psychology,* 1949, *19,* 210-219.

Keogh, B. K., Vernon, M., & Smith, C. E. Deafness and visual-motor functions. *Journal of Special Education,* 1970, *4*(1), 41-47.

Levine, E. S. Studies in psychological evaluation of the deaf. *Volta Review,* 1963, *65*(9), 496-511.

Levine, E. S. Mental assessment of the deaf child. *Volta Review,* 1971, *73*(2), 80-105.

Levine, E. S. Psychological tests and practices with the deaf: A survey of the state of the art. *Volta Review,* 1974, *76*(5), 298-319.

Levine, E. S. Psychological evaluation of the deaf client. In B. Bolton (Ed.), *Handbook of measurement and evaluation in rehabilitation.* Baltimore: University Park Press, 1976.

Levine, E. (Ed.). The preparation of psychological service providers to the deaf. *Journal of Rehabilitation of the Deaf,* Monograph No. 4, 1977.

Levine, E. S. *The ecology of early deafness: Guides to fashioning environments and psychological assessments.* New York: Columbia University Press, 1981.

Lyon, V. W. Personality tests with the deaf. *American Annals of the Deaf,* 1934, *79*(1), 1-4.

Lyon V. W. The use of vocational and personality tests with the deaf. *Journal of Applied Psychology,* 1934, *18,* 224-230.

Meadow, K. P. Personality and social development of deaf persons. *Journal of Rehabilitation of the Deaf,* 1976, *9*(3), 1-12.

Myklebust, H. R. *Auditory disorders in children: A manual for differential diagnosis.* New York: Grune & Stratton, 1954.

Myklebust, H. R. *The psychology of deafness: Sensory deprivation, learning, and adjustment* (2nd ed.). New York: Grune & Stratton, 1964.

Osler, S. P. The nature of intelligence. *Volta Review,* 1965, *67*(4), 285-291.

Pintner, R., Fusfeld, I., & Brunschwig, L. Personality tests of deaf adults. *Journal of Genetic Psychology,* 1937, *51,* 305-327.

Quendenfield, C., & Bartkiw, N. Life style analyses: A method for assessing the deaf client. *Journal of Rehabilitation of the Deaf,* 1980, *14*(2), 8-13.

Reamer, J. C. Mental and educational measurements of the deaf. *Psychological Monographs,* 1921, *29*(132).

Rosenstein, J. Social and vocational assessment. *Volta Review,* 1963, *65*(9), 542-547.

Ross, A. O. *Psychological aspects of learning disabilities and reading disorders.* New York: McGraw-Hill, 1976.

Sachs, B., Trybus, R. J., Koch, H., & Falberg, R. M. Current developments in the psychological evaluation of deaf individuals. *Journal of Rehabilitation of the Deaf,* 1974, *8*(1), 131-141.

Sanderson, R. Preparation of the hearing impaired for an adult vocational life. *Journal of Rehabilitation of the Deaf,* 1973, *6*(3), 12-18.

Schick, H. F. A performance test for deaf children of school age. *Volta Review,* 1934, *36,* 657-658.

Sullivan, P. M., & Vernon, M. Psychological assessment of hearing-impaired children. *School Psychology Digest,* 1979, *8*(3), 271-290.

Vernon, M. A guide to psychological tests and testing procedures in the evaluation of deaf and hard-of-hearing children. *Journal of Speech and Hearing Disorders,* 1964, *29*(4), 414-423.

Vernon, M. A guide for the psychological evaluation of deaf and severely hard-of-hearing adults. *The Deaf American,* 1967, *19*(9), 15-18.

Vernon, M. Fifty years of research on the intelligence of deaf and hard-of-hearing children: A review of literature and discussion of implications. *Journal of Rehabilitation of the Deaf*, 1968, *1*(4), 1-12.

Vernon, M. Psychological evaluation of the severely handicapped deaf client. In L. Stewart (Ed.), *Toward more effective rehabilitation services for the severely handicapped deaf client*. Little Rock: Arkansas Rehabilitation Research and Training Center, 1971.

Vernon, M., Bair, R., & Lotz, S. Psychological evaluation and testing of children who are deaf-blind. *School Psychology Digest*, 1979, *8*(3), 291-295.

Vernon, M., & Brown, D. W. A guide to psychological tests and testing procedures in the evaluation of deaf and hard-of-hearing children. *Journal of Speech and Hearing Disorders*, 1964, *29*(4), 414-423.

Vernon, M., & Green, D. A guide to the psychological assessment of deaf-blind adults. *Journal of Visual Impairment & Blindness*, 74 (June 1980), 229-231.

Vollenweidner, J. A. Psychological testing. In J. D. Rainer & K. Z. Altshuler (Eds.), *Psychiatry and the deaf: Report of the workshop for psychiatrists on extending mental health services to the deaf*. New York: New York University (Center for Research and Training in Deafness Rehabilitation), 1967.

Watson, D. (Ed.). *Deaf evaluation and adjustment feasibility*. New York: New York University (Deafness Research and Training Center), 1976.

APPENDIX B

TEST ACRONYMS

Acronym	Test	Page
BMCT	Bennett Mechanical Comprehension Tests	87
BSAB	Balthazar Scales of Adaptive Behavior I & II	55
BVRT	Benton Visual Retention Test	79
CIIS	Cattell Infant Intelligence Scale	25
CMMS	Columbia Mental Maturity Scale	27
CPI	California Psychological Inventory	57
CTP	California Test of Personality	58
DABRS	Devereux Adolescent Behavior Rating Scale	60
DAP	Draw-a-Person Projective Technique	61
DAT	Differential Aptitude Test	89
DDST	Denver Developmental Screening Test	29
DSCF	Denver Scale of Communication Function	21
FIT	Flanagan Industrial Tests	91
FDT	O'Conner Finger Dexterity Test	99
FRPVT	Full-Range Picture Vocabulary Test	5
GAPSP	Grace Arthur Point Scale of Performance	34
GATB	General Aptitude Test Battery	92
GCT	General Clerical Test	94
GPII	Geist Picture Interest Inventory	105
GPII:D:M	Geist Picture Interest Inventory: Deaf: Male	106
GMRT	Gates-MacGinitie Reading Tests	7
HIS	Haptic Intelligence Scale for Adult Blind	30
HPI	Handicap Problems Inventory	63
H-NTLA	Hiskey-Nebraska Test of Learning Aptitude	32
H-T-P	House-Tree-Person Projective Technique	64
ITPA	Illinois Test of Psycholinguistic Abilities	23
JEVS	Jewish Employment and Vocational Service	115
KBDT	Kohs Block Design Test	36
KCT	Knox Cube Test: Arthur Revision	34
LIPS	Leiter International Performance Scale	37
MAT	Metropolitan Achievement Tests Series	10
MCT	Minnesota Clerical Test	96
MFD	Memory for Designs Test	81
MMPI	Minnesota Multiphasic Personality Inventory	68

Acronym	Test	Page
MPFB-R	Revised Minnesota Paper Form Board Test	102
MRMT	Minnesota Rate of Manipulation Tests	97
MVPT	Motor-Free Visual Perception Test	83
NATB	Nonreading Aptitude Test Battery	93
PIES	Picture Interest Exploration Survey	108
PPVT	Peabody Picture Vocabulary Test	12
RBE	Revised Beta Examination	39
R-INT	Reitan-Indiana Neuropsychological Test Battery for Children	84
RPM	Raven's Progressive Matrices	42
SAT-HI	Stanford Achievement Test—Hearing-Impaired Edition	14
S-BIS	Stanford-Binet Intelligence Scale	44
SCII	Strong-Campbell Interest Inventory	109
SEAI	Meadow/Kendall Social-Emotional Assessment Inventory	66
SIT	Slosson Intelligence Test	40
SVES	Singer Vocational Evaluation System	117
TAT	Thematic Apperception Test	74
TDT	O'Conner Tweezer Dexterity Test	99
TOWER	Testing, Orientation and Work Evaluation in Rehabilitation	119
TSCS	Tennessee Self Concept Scale	72
VCWSS	Valpar Component Work Sample Series	120
VLDS	Verbal Language Development Scale	16
VSMS	Vineland Social Maturity Scale	46
WAIS-R	Wechsler Adult Intelligence Scale—Revised	48
WISC-R	Wechsler Intelligence Scale for Children—Revised	50
WPPSI	Wechsler Preschool and Primary Scale of Intelligence	50
WRAT	Wide Range Achievement Test	18
WRIOT-R	Wide Range Interest and Opinion Test—Revised	111
WRMT	Woodcock Reading Mastery Tests	19

Frank Zieziula is an associate professor in the Department of Counseling of Gallaudet College's School of Education and Human Services. A native of Buffalo, New York, he received his doctor of philosophy degree in counselor education from New York University. He worked with hearing-impaired people for four years at the National Technical Institute for the Deaf, Rochester, N.Y., and for five years at the New York University Deafness Research and Training Center, New York City, before coming to Gallaudet College in 1977. His published works have appeared in the *American Annals of the Deaf*, the *Journal of Rehabilitation of the Deaf*, and the *Personnel and Guidance Journal*.